AF553205

CHILD DEVELOPMENT

Child Development

Issues and Country Experiences

Edited by

Anusri Mallik

2012

Icfai Books
The Icfai University Press

CHILD DEVELOPMENT: ISSUES AND COUNTRY EXPERIENCES

Editor: Anusri Mallik

First Edition: 2012
Printed in India

Published by

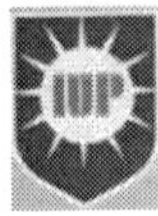

This book is published by IUP.
University Campus, Agartala-Simna Road,
P.O. Kamalghat Sadar, Agartala – 799210, Tripura (West)
E-mail: info@iupindia.org
Website: www.books.iupindia.org

ISBN: 978-81-314-2710-1

Contents

SECTION II

COUNTRY EXPERIENCES

Overview

Child development refers to the biological and psychological changes that occur in human beings between birth and the end of adolescence, as the individual progresses from dependency to increasing autonomy. It is a complex process. Therefore, an understanding of the various influences on child development and how they interact is crucial to the design of successful interventions. Developmental change may occur as a result of genetically-controlled processes known as maturation, or as a result of environmental factors and learning, but most commonly involves an interaction between the two. The optimal development of children is considered vital to society and so it is important to understand the social, cognitive, emotional and educational development of children. Increased research and interest in this field has resulted in new theories and strategies, with specific regard to practice that promotes development within the school system.

Childhood is the base of any society. A child's 'growth' depends on nutrition, health, education and in the final count, financial support from

Government or NGOs. Statistics show that children living in abject poverty, in fragile economic and social environment are those whose physical and mental development are most challenged. According to the World Development Report (2008), 16% of under-fives suffered from underweight due to lack of nutrition in South Asia (10% of under-fives in developing countries as a whole) and 77% of under-fives suffer from suspected pneumonia in South Asia (69% of under-fives in developing countries as a whole) per annum.

The early development of cognitive skills, emotional well-being, social competence and sound physical and mental health builds a strong foundation for success well into the adult years. Beyond their short-term importance for positive school achievement, these abilities are critical prerequisites for economic productivity and responsible citizenship throughout life. All aspects of adult human capital, from work-force skills to cooperative and lawful behavior, build on capacities which are developed during childhood, beginning at birth.

The basic principles of neuroscience and the process of human skill formation indicate that early intervention for the most vulnerable children will generate the greatest payback. Although the large number of children and families who could benefit from additional assistance will require significant increases in funding, extensive research indicates that investment in high quality interventions will generate substantial future returns through increased taxes paid by more productive adults and significant reductions in public expenditures for special education, grade retention, welfare assistance and incarceration. Stated simply, the largest returns will be realized from effective services for the neediest children and families well before they enter school.

This book is divided into two sections. Section I "**Introduction**" provides basic concepts and some related issues of child development. The introductory article of this section, "**Child Development: An Overview**" is written by *Anusri Mallik*. The article reveals that many children younger than 5 years in developing countries are exposed to multiple risks, including poverty, malnutrition, poor health and unstimulating home environments, which detrimentally affect their cognitive, motor, social and emotional development. These are the basic indicators of development of young children in developing countries. Most of these children live in south Asia and sub-Saharan Africa. These disadvantaged children are likely to do poorly in school. In later childhood, these children will subsequently have poor levels of cognition and education, both of which are linked to later earnings. The failure of children to fulfill their developmental potential and to achieve satisfactory educational levels plays an important part in the intergenerational transmission of poverty. The study of child development or child psychology teaches parents to plan activities and experiences for their children and to take proper care of their children by developing a proper understanding with them which fulfill their needs. Child psychology studies the behaviour of the child in all situations such as home, school and community and also explains how a child passes through various stages of growth and gives an idea about the characteristics of each stage. The teacher or parents can have knowledge of the pattern of development of a child. For example, memory for concrete objects develops during the early years, whereas memory for abstract materials develops in the late years. The power of learning is highest in the early years. The study of child development gives detailed knowledge about the relationship of heredity and environment which are both responsible for human growth and development. The child gets his mental and physical qualities from his parents, but development of these qualities is affected by the environment. In the paper, an attempt has been made to provide an overview of child development with available worldwide data.

The second article titled, **"What Matters for Child Development?"** is contributed by *Fali Huang*. The main aim of the paper is to estimate early child cognitive and social development results. Since home and school inputs are often endogenous choices of parents and hence are correlated with each other and across periods, any omitted inputs would necessarily cause bias in estimated effects of included ones. To minimize the omitted variable problem, the paper adopts various within-child differences and value-added specifications to deal with the unobserved family and child fixed factors, and uses a comprehensive set of detailed inputs. A small subset of inputs is found consistently important in explaining variances of child development results, including the number of books a child has at various ages and how often a mother reads to a child by age five, while the effects of race and maternal employment are negligible when detailed inputs are controlled. The paper shows that the racial gaps of math and reading scores among eight and nine year-old children can be completely accounted for by home and school inputs. The estimation results in various specifications yielding a consistent picture, where a reasonably small set of earlier and current inputs are important predictors for child development results at age eight or nine. The number of books a child has at various ages and how often a mother reads to her child before age 5 are the most important predictors of child math and reading scores from age five onwards; they are also primary predictors of child behavior problem scores at age 5. Spanking a child aged 8-9 seems to be mostly driven by family or child fixed factors while spanking a younger child may reduce his future behavior problems. When detailed home and school inputs are controlled, a mother's working hours in the first five years of a child's life have little effects on child aged at 8-9.

The next article titled as "**Child Health: Concepts and Issues**" is written by *Dalia Dey* and *Kasturi Nandy*. The article states that health has a major effect on the strength of body and mind and the cognitive development of the child. A healthy and productive child can contribute to the workforce which adds value to the overall economic growth of a nation. The Millennium Development Goal (MDG) (Goal 4), aims to reduce child mortality rate among children under five by two-thirds between 1990 and 2015. Proper sanitation measures, clean surroundings, hygienic living conditions are required for total development of a child, which have been discussed in the article. The article also reflects industrialization and its effect on child health. Besides economic conditions, race and gender have a major stake in the case of child health and overall development. Finally, the steps which have been taken globally for overall development of the children and few interventions by some international organizations like WHO, UNICEF have been discussed in the article. Experts are engaged in identifying the factors which are hindrances to the proper growth of a child. Apart from the income, which ensures the availability of adequate food, health care and nutrition are few essential elements which a child requires for his balanced growth. The environment, in which a child grows up, is also one of the most influential elements. Other elements, which according to experts, have a contributory role towards the total development of a child are – proper sanitation measures, clean surroundings, hygienic living conditions etc. Parental education surely has a relation to the financial establishment of a family. A family, consisting of educated parents, is more likely to have a modest income, which, in turn, ensures the availability of adequate nutritious food. Also, the educated parents are expected to have more knowledge about healthy food habits, balanced diet, hygiene, proper sanitation measures, immunization measures available and the preventive measures to be taken for their child. Possibility of gender discrimination, being practiced mostly among illiterate segment of society, is expected to be low in educated families and hence it leads to healthier outcome in terms of proper birth spacing and number of children. Educated parents are expected to develop healthy food habits in their children to prevent the problems of obesity.

The fourth article titled, "**Behaviour Development in Babies: Its Improvement in Relation with Ecological Factors**" is contributed by *Bimla Dhanda* and *Sudha Chhikara*. The article shows that the infants' early interaction experiences are determined by a multitude of biological, cultural and environmental factors. If the performance of an infant in a particular development is declining it may be improved by improving his home environment or the enforcement by an intervention programme. In view of these points, present investigation was undertaken with the aim of identifying the developmental deficiencies in babies with reference to social skill development, delineating the crucial ecological factors affecting this development and studying the impact of intervention programme on social skill development. The study was conducted at two locations, viz., Hisar city as urban and Rawalwas Klan and Siswal villages as rural. The purposes of selection of localities were easy accessibility and rapport with the respondents. In social skill development, males, in general, were better than females. Interaction of age and gender also revealed that the boys learned social skills differently than girls over the different age groups. Comparison of urban and rural sample also revealed that urban babies, in general, were better than rural ones in social skill development. Regarding associations with economic factors, it appeared that the babies from higher income group generally had better development in social skills under both urban and rural areas. Intervention proved highly effective for development of social skills in both urban and rural areas.

The fifth article "**Malnutrition and the Developing Mind**" is written by *Bhoomika Rastogi Kar, Shobini L Rao* and *B A Chandramouli*. The article deals about the nutritional deficiency which can disrupt the structure and function of the nervous system of humans. Malnutrition is associated with both structural and functional pathology of the brain. Structurally malnutrition results in tissue damage, growth retardation, disorderly differentiation, reduction in synapses and synaptic neurotransmitters, delayed myelination and reduced overall development of dendritic arborization of the developing brain. Malnutrition affects brain and cognitive development. Developing mind is sensitive to the effects of brain damage caused by malnutrition. There are deviations in the temporal sequences of brain maturation, which in turn disturb the formation of neuronal circuits.

Brain development and cognitive maturation occur concurrently during childhood and adolescence. Developmental neuro imaging has provided data on postnatal structural and functional maturation of the brain-from childhood to adolescence. Structural maturation of brain regions and connections determine cognitive development to a certain extent. However, less clear-cut relationships have been observed between development of brain structure and cognitive development. Its continues to undergo major changes after birth—throughout childhood and adolescence. Its growth is marked by neuro developmental events such as neuronal density, dendritic growth, synaptic density and myelination. Cortical changes between childhood and adolescence are confined to dorsal regions prominently frontal and parietal cortices, which are related to improved cognitive abilities. Brain growth occurs in spurts showing a change at irregular intervals approximately every two years. Myelination is a neuro developmental event, which continues until adolescence and shows different rates of maturation across different brain regions. Ongoing process of myelination is related to the formation of networks and development of higher cognitive functions during childhood and adolescence.

The subsequent article "**Beyond Quality in Early Childhood Education and Care – Languages of Evaluation**" is contributed by *Peter Moss* and *Gunilla Dahlberg*. This paper views that every product and service must offer quality and every consumer wants to have it. It is an essential attribute of services or products that gives them value. The problem with quality, from this perspective, is its management. The paper discusses how quality can be discovered, measured, assured and improved and what goals, to be achieved by technical means, will enhance performance and increase value. Further, it highlights the work of well trained staffs who are committed to work with children for development and improvement of quality. Also, the staffs ensure continuity, stability and developmentally appropriate curriculum with educational content for the overall development of the children. The paper also describes the current expansion of early childhood education and care which provides, potentially, many benefits and possibilities for children, parents and wider society. The authors opine that expansion brings with it major risks, which are increasing regulation and normalisation, what Nikolas Rose terms "governing the soul". If these risks are to be reduced and the potential benefits are to be realized, societies need to put technical and managerial practice in place, as subservient to democratic political and ethical practice, and to open themselves to diversity and experimentation.

The seventh article titled, "**Parenting and Responsibility: Holding Parents Accountable for Children's Antisocial Practices**" is written by *E A Uwe*, *P N Asuquo* and *E E Ekuri*. The crux of the paper is as follows: proper nurturing of children is the primary responsibility of parents. Parents have inescapable responsibilities when bringing up their children. These responsibilities are automatically conferred on both parents of the child right from the child's birth. They are expected to guide and modify the behaviour of their child to conform to the acceptable behaviours in the society as well as participate in activities aimed at preventing crime or disorder being committed by children. Ironically, some parents have failed in these roles and functions. They are too permissive and adopt laissez-faire parenting style that inadvertently makes their children vulnerable to anti-social behaviours. Some parents are hostile, indifferent and rarely show affection to their children. They neglect or beat their children, but rarely exercise consistent firm guidance. Some are so permissive that they do not care about what happens to their children, or what they do. Such parents produce delinquent children. Furthermore, in permissive homes, children get premature autonomy. They come and go as they wish. With such inconsistent parents, children become relatively confused as to the reactions they would get. The paper focuses on parents as the catalysts for children's behaviour. The rationale for children's anti-social behaviours is highlighted as well as some of the corrupt behaviours parents exhibit. The root causes of these behaviours are brought to limelight and suggestions proffered for improving the task of parenting.

Section II – Experiences explores some country studies. It begins with the article "**Intra-Urban and Intra-Rural Inequities in Child Health: Evidence from Sub-Saharan Africa**" which is contributed by *Jean-Christophe Fotso*. Over the last few decades, sub-Saharan Africa has witnessed an urban population explosion despite poor macroeconomic performance, making it difficult for national and urban authorities to provide affordable housing, quality social services, or sufficient employment to the growing urban populations. Recent estimates indicate that about 42% of the urban population in most sub-Saharan African countries live in "life and health threatening" homes or neighborhoods. On the other hand, improvements in child survival have been very poor in the region, and progress in child nutritional well-being observed worldwide continues to bypass many African countries and population subgroups. Against the foregoing backdrop, the paper seeks to revisit the urban advantage in health by examining differences across urban and rural areas in health inequalities. Specifically, its goal is to compare the magnitude of inequities in child malnutrition across urban and rural areas; and compare the intra-urban inequities with urban-rural differences. The paper suggests that failing to appropriately target the growing sub-group of the urban poor and improve their living conditions and health status, policies and programs geared at improving children's welfare, including the MDGs, may not meet their national goals. In addition to improving the overall urban and national averages of health indicators, it is important to analyze, track and purposefully reduce health inequities, since progress towards the achievement of the health MDGs will not automatically benefit the underprivileged population sub-groups.

The next article titled, **"What Ails the Children of this World? – Some Evidences from Latin America and the Caribbean"** is written by *Paramita Mookherjee Nag*. The article points out that young children in many developing countries suffer from profound deficits in nutrition, health, fine and gross motor skills, cognitive development and socio-emotional development. Early Childhood Development (ECD) outcomes are important markers of the welfare of children in their own right. In addition, the deleterious effects of poor outcomes in early childhood can be long-lasting, affecting school attainment, employment, wages, criminality and measures of social integration of adults. This article considers the theoretical case to be made for investments in early childhood, selectively reviews the literature on the impact of ECD programs in the United States, discusses the evidence from Latin America and the Caribbean and makes suggestions for future research. According to economic theories it is expected that there would be high returns if investments are made in early childhood. Making up the deficiencies in the cognitive and non-cognitive behaviour later in life incurs a higher cost and is more often than not prohibitive and unsuccessful. In contrast, it is found that investing in preschool programs has a higher sense of success and a greater impact among preschool children. In Latin American and the Caribbean, any idea of the relationship between poverty, illiteracy, malnutrition, various socio-economic parameters and child development programs and policies is found to be disappointingly lax. Yet there are some opinions, after analyzing the data, that the economic costs incurred due to the lack of cognitive and non cognitive abilities in the Caribbean and the Latin America are as large as or even larger than that estimated for United States. The focus is on the relation between outcomes in early childhood and measures of household socioeconomic status, child health, and parenting practices, as well as on the impact of specific policies and programs. The knowledge base on early childhood outcomes is still thin in Latin America and the Caribbean. There are therefore very high returns to comparative descriptive analysis in the region, as well as to careful evaluations of the impact of various programs.

The next article **"Early Childhood Development and Social Mobility"** is contributed by *Barnett, W Steven* and *Belfield, Clive R.* This paper examines the effects of preschool education on social mobility in the United States. The authors note that under the current policy, three- and four-year-old children from economically and educationally disadvantaged families have higher preschool attendance rates than other children. Increased investment in preschool, conclude Barnett and Belfield, could raise social mobility. Program expansions targeted to disadvantaged children would help them move up the ladder, as would a more universal set of policies from which disadvantaged children could gain disproportionately. To them educational effectiveness of early childhood programs would provide for greater gains in social mobility than increasing participation rates alone. The authors observe that if future expansions of preschool programs end up serving all children, not just the poorest, society as a whole would gain. Benefits would exceed costs and there would be more economic growth, but relative gains for disadvantaged children would be smaller than absolute gains because there would be some (smaller) benefits to other children. Investments in the skills of a nation's citizens can affect both the general level of their productivity and income and disparities in incomes and living standards among them. The paper examines how current public investments in preschool education for US children are affecting the skills of those children, generally, as well as the extent to which the investments are reducing income-related disparities among them—not only during childhood but also when they are adults. The authors also consider how new investments in those programs might affect children's skills and increase social mobility.

The final article "**Child Labour and Child Right to Education in South Asia with Particular Reference to India and Bangladesh**" is written by *Anusri Mallik*. According to the paper, the twin issues of child labour and children's rights to education have become a matter of international concern while gaining prominence in national developmental efforts. Within the South Asian context, the issue of child labour is widely seen as a manifestation of poverty, and the child's contribution to the household economy is seen as vital to meeting the basic needs of poor families. This region has the largest number of child labourers in the world, as well as the largest number of children out of school. The paper explores the nature of the conflict between the right of the child to education and the economic needs of the family and which of these concerns should take priority. The need for education in relation to certain sections of the population which include women, scheduled castes, schedule tribes and other backward classes in India is important to rectify ancient inequities in a family and society. Demographers and economists have pointed to the links between female literacy, lower fertility rates and improved welfare of the society. Children have both the right to education and the need for education. Being pragmatic about the need to work and opposing the right to education, one is opposing an inter-generational perspective at all. Indeed one is falling into the trap of taking the existing reality as given. We all know that poverty is not a given phenomenon. Several factors like colonialism, capitalism, wrong government policy etc. are responsible for it. Nowadays in many countries, poverty has declined due to suitable public policy, effective public action, satisfactory economic growth rate and targeted initiatives. Even when poverty has not reduced, explanations can be traced to the nature of economy and polity. People in or on the margins frequently swing to above the poverty line, though this depends to a great extent on how much below the line they originally were. Poverty then, is not static or immobile at any fixed point in time. The paper also discusses the role of the state in this context. Finally, it highlights the status of child labour in the context of globalization and international trade agreements and brings together a range of perspectives concerning the causes of and solutions to the problem of child labour in South Asia.

Section I

Introduction

1

Child Development: An Overview

Anusri Mallik

Development of the child can be defined as the emergence and expansion of his/her capacities to provide greater facility in functioning. To some extent this development is measured in four major terms namely anatomic, cognitive, behavioural and social development. In developing countries, a large number of children are suffering from multiple risks including extreme poverty, malnutrition, ill health, illiteracy, unstimulating and unhealthy home atmosphere. These factors detrimentally affect their development. In this paper an attempt has been made to provide an overview of child development with available worldwide data.

Introduction

Development of the child can be defined as the emergence and expansion of his/her capacities to provide greater facility in functioning. This development is achieved through the process of growth, maturation and learning which has two aspects of change: one is quantity and the other is quality.

Development is achieved through the processes of growth which refers to quantitative change in size and structure. It also refers to an increase in magnitude – in body size, in muscular strength, and in intellectual ability. It consists of a progressive series of changes of an orderly coherent type towards the goal of maturity. We can also say development is more than a concept which can be observed, appraised and to some extent measured in four major terms – anatomic, cognitive, behavioural and social development.

Development of physical and mental traits of the individual comes partly from an intrinsic maturity of those traits and partly from exercises and experiences that he undergoes. Growth is a measure of physical maturation. It signifies an increase in the size of the body and its different organs. A serious disturbance of growth may affect the development of the brain resulting in delay in the acquisition of skills like writing, social adaptation and speech.

Human beings are never static. From the moment of conception until death, the individual is constantly changing in all developmental contexts. There are certain features which are characteristic of human development and which influence greatly the form it takes. Growth and development follow certain principles:

(1) Development follows a Pattern

Every species, whether animal or human, follows a pattern of development peculiar to their species, and the rate and limits of development are similar for all members of the species. In the case of human beings, development is in an orderly pattern. The relatively helpless, unskilled, uncontrolled infant achieves the succession of development tasks by an orderly sequence of acquisitions.

(2) Every Individual Normally Passes through Each Major Stage of Development :

Each stage has certain characteristics some of which stand out more conspicuously than others. Since there are individual differences in the rate of growth, age limits for different stages can be regarded as merely approximate and suggestive. However, the entire period of development is divided into the following stages:

(a) Pre-natal period : From conception to birth

(b) Neo-natal stage : From birth to two weeks

(c) Infancy : From two weeks to one year

(d) Babyhood : From one year to two years

(e) Childhood : From two to twelve years

(f) Adolescence : From thirteen onwards

(3) Development Proceeds from General to Specific Response

In all phases of development, whether motor or mental, the child's responses are of a general nature before they become specific. In both prenatal and postnatal development general activity precedes specific ones.

(4) Development is Continuous

There is no discontinuity in development. It is a continuous process from the moment of conception to death.

(5) Individual differences in rate of development remain constant

There is plenty of evidence to show that the rate of growth is constant. Those who develop rapidly at first will continue to do so, while those whose development was slow will develop slowly. For example, curves of heights have shown that children who are tall at one age are tall at other ages also, while those who are short remain short.

(6) The rate of development is different for different parts of the body

Not all parts of the body grow at the same rate, nor do all aspects of mental growth proceed equally. The different phases of mental and physical growth occur at their own individual rates and reach maturity at different times. In some areas of the body, the growth is rapid, while in others, the growth may be slow. Thus, the pattern of relative size of the organs of the body changes from time to time.

(7) Most traits are co-related in development:

The popular assumption that compensation is a general rule in the development of a child is not borne out by experimental studies. It is not true that the child who is above average in one trait will be below average in others, as a means of equalizing his capacities. The rate of development for different parts of the body differs, but they are compensatory in the above average growth in height during one period which may be accompanied by below average growth in weight. Gsell observed that there is a relationship between the development of physical and mental traits. Development of language, for example, is related to the development of speech organs. It is difficult to find someone who is above average in one trait but below the normal in another trait. Genetic studies have shown that desired traits go together.

(8) Development is predictable

Since the rate of development for each child is constant, it is possible to predict at an early age the range within which the mature development of the child is likely to fall. It will be knowing what the ultimate mental development of a child will be is of outstanding value in the planning of his education and helps him to train himself for the type of work he is best suited to carry out.

(9) Each development phase has traits-characteristic of its own

At each age, some traits develop more rapidly and more conspicuously than others. Each stage of development is distinguished by a dominant feature, a leading characteristic, which gives the period its coherence and unity. Up to the age of 2 years, for example, the baby concentrates on his environment, growing control over his body and learning to speak. From the age of 3-6 years his development is concentrated on making him a more social creature.

(10) Many forms of so called "Problem Behaviour" are normal behaviour of the age in which they occur

Every age has certain undesirable forms of behaviour which are normally found at that age and are outgrown as the child passes onto the next stage of development. For example, lying is a common mode of behaviour which is manifested when the child enters the school. Similarly, day-dreaming is quite normal in early stages of school. Hence, the child's behaviour is to be predicted and understood against the expected behaviour of his age.

(11) Individual differences exist in development

All children do not reach the same point of development at the same speed at the same age. Some children differ in their rate of development, going through the sequential steps as expected, but at a slower or faster rate than average children. Thus, there are "slow growers" and "fast growers". These differences are influenced both by hereditary potentials and environmental factors. For example, all the children have the same organs, the same body constituents, the same functions but in all instances differ in some degree in both structure and functioning of these organs.

Need and Importance of the Study of Child Development:

Every individual grows through many changes. His opinions, attitudes and aspirations undergo continuous changes.

The study of child development or child psychology teaches parents to plan activities and experiences for their children and to take proper care of their children by developing a proper understanding with them which fulfill their needs.

Child psychology studies the behaviour of the child in all situations such as home, school and community and also explains how a child passes through various stages of growth and gives an idea about the characteristics of each stage.

The teacher or parents can have knowledge of the pattern of development of a child. For example, memory for concrete objects develops during the early years, whereas memory for abstract materials develops in the late years. The power of learning is highest in the early years.

The study of child development gives detailed knowledge about the relationship of heredity and environment which are both responsible for human growth and development. The child gets his mental and physical qualities from his parents, but development of these qualities is affected by his environment.

Child development also explains problem behaviour of children which are expected at various stages and suggests various ways to handle these. Thus, a mother can identify and understand better what behaviour is the characteristic behaviour and what behaviour is the problem behaviour of the child. Furthermore, it provides knowledge about the nutritional pattern and nutritional needs of the children. The parent-child relationship is one of the most important factors of child development. Many individuals in society show evidence of maladjustment and serious emotional disturbance, causes of which lie in unhealthy relationship between parents and children.

In addition to the above knowledge, child psychology is important for every individual as it gives additional information about character formation of the child, his personality development, health and sanitary rules, simple diseases that affect the child and immunization to develop the child into a healthy and balanced youth.

Areas of Development

I. Physical Development

Physical development can be defined as the series of anatomic and physiological changes taking place between the beginning of pre-natal life and senility. It denotes change in size, quality and quantity. Motor Development is also associated with physical growth and proceeds in general, from head to foot. For example, the baby first lifts his head from a surface and later he moves arms, shoulders and abdominal muscles.

Changes in Height, Weight and Shape

Changes in Height

The height of the newborn is one-third of the final height, and by the end of the second year the child gains about half of his total height. At the time of birth, the child measures about 19-20 inches in height and in one year his height increases to about 30 inches. In the second year, 5 inches are added to his height. After this, child gains about 2-2.5 inches every year until adolescence.

From birth through the period of growth, boys and girls differ in the amount and pattern of physical growth. Girls are generally more mature than boys of the same age. The period of 'spurt' starts around 10-11 years for girls and 12-13 years for boys. The growth during this time is less intense for girls and lasts for a shorter period than the boys' adolescent spurt. During this time boys will add an average of about 8 inches to their height, while girls will add an average of about 6.5 inches. Girls' physical growth is steady and more predictable than that of boys.

Change in Weight

The average weight of newborns varies between 6-8 pounds. In the 4-6 months after birth infants double their birth-weight and by the end of the first year, the birth weight is tripled; by the end of the second year, the birth weight is quadrupled and after this there is steady increase of about 5 to 6 pounds per year.

The weight of boys is more in infancy and childhood as compared to girls. During the period of 'spurt' boys gain about 45 pounds of weight while girls gain approximately 35 pounds. Weight gain is influenced by exercise and disease.

Change in Other Body Parts

Although growth in the first half year after birth is rapid, changes in body proportion are relatively slight. The hands, feet, arms and legs are much longer or larger in proportion to the rest of the body. The head to body length ratio also changes from 1:4 at infancy to 1:7.5 at adulthood; lower limbs change from 1:3 for infants to 1:2 for adults.

Skeleton structure, musculature and distribution of fat also change markedly during the growth and maturation process. The bones harden at different rates. Enhanced hardening rate is found in the bones of hand and wrist. Hand and foot growth is faster at first, followed by increase in growth rate of calf, forearm, hips, chest, shoulders, trunk and depth of chest. In males, from puberty to maturity, growth of the trunk and limbs is at first equal, followed by a relatively rapid growth of trunk later. In females, from puberty to maturity, the trunk develops in the lumber region and the pelvis enlarges. The most important factor influencing physical development is nutrition. Malnourished or undernourished children will not have average height. Certain diseases also interrupt normal growth of height and weight. The amount of exercise and socio-emotional adjustment will also affect height and weight growth. Children brought up in homes where there is a great deal of emotional stress may show hampered growth rate. In many cases, bright children are larger than dull children and reach puberty slightly earlier.

II. Motor Development

The most important development of children in the first year is the development of the ability to control many muscles and the co-ordination of different maturing systems. At birth children are helpless to the extent that they cannot move their body and are unable to grasp anything placed near them. By the end of the first year they are able to co-ordinate different parts of their body and control their different muscles.

Many studies have shown that this control follows an orderly pattern. Motor performances involving arms, wrists and fingers such as reaching, grasping and thumb opposition develop in a sequence. Motor ability of the child helps him to cope with his environment and modifies his physical health.

Factors affecting Motor Development

i) Individual Differences

The age for maturation for each individual is different and this difference creates individuality in motor development. Most of the children crawl before they walk, however, some walk before they crawl and the ages at which the children enter the various developmental stages may also vary.

ii) Sex

In infancy there are no sex differences in activity level. These differences develop when children attain the age of social play. For example, boys are encouraged to play with blocks or to do woodwork while girls are encouraged to indulge in more passive activities.

iii) Fantasy

A child's fantasy life plays an important role in motor development. Many motor skills are learnt during play activities which have imaginative content, for example, doll play and housekeeping.

iv) Culture

According to many researchers culture plays a crucial role in motor development. To them there is difference in age at which various skills are attained in different societies. For example, hunters succeed in rearing infants who walk earlier and run faster.

v) Intelligence

The relationship between intelligence and motor development, specially during the first year of life is important. Babies who are extremely slow in sitting, standing or walking generally prove to be backward in intellectual development. The age of walking, in particular has been found to be associated with intelligence.

vi) Poor Physical Condition

There is a close relationship between the physical condition of a child and motor development. It has been proved that the child with superior health is more precocious in motor development than the child whose physical condition is poor. It is seen that the child with poor health gets less opportunity for exercise and physical activities. This is likely to make children more backward.

III. Emotional Development

Emotional development is related with cognitive/behavioural development. Every child is born with the potential for emotional expression. Emotion is a label for a vast range of psychosomatic states which involve feeling, perception or awareness of an event or circumstance. The word emotion covers condition of both positive and negative character. The condition in which an individual is eager, zestful, jubilant and moved up is referred to as a positive condition, while on the other hand, the condition in which an individual feels disturbed, distressed and moved away or against is referred to as a negative condition. In psychology negative emotion is treated primarily as a form of disorder and distress.

The most common childhood emotions are fear, anger, jealousy, joy and pleasure, love and affection etc. All emotions play a crucial role in child's life, each contributing to the social and personal adjustment of the individual. The child is capable of profound emotional expression even before birth. At the time of birth the child has simple emotions but as he grows overtime, more complex emotions are developed through maturation and learning. A newborn's emotions are diffused and lack in differentiation. By the end of the first year the baby develops fear, anger, jealousy, envy, curiosity, joy and affection. The number of emotional reactions is dependent upon age. Negative reactions predominate in the second half of the first year of life while the positive reactions are highest at the age of three.

Importance of Childhood Emotions

An emotion represents effective feeling tones in which the whole body takes part. An individual is not born with any set of emotional expressions. These attitudes and feelings are developed as he grows up and have a profound effect upon the way he reacts to any situation. Both positive and negative types of emotions are important for children.

i) Emotions affect social interaction

Child learns to modify his/her behaviour and acquires knowledge about social standards and expectations from different patterns of emotional behaviour. Some negative expressions like anger and jealousy encourage unpleasant social interaction while joy, happiness, love and affection encourage pleasant social interaction.

ii) Emotions add pleasure to everyday experience

The after effect of positive emotions gives pleasure to the children. For example, emotions like joy, pleasure, love and affection leads them to a positive direction.

iii) Emotions serve as social communicator

The child can articulate his feelings for a person or for a particular situation by changing his bodily and facial expressions.

iv) Emotions serve as self-evaluator

The maturity of the child can be evaluated by observing his reactions and expressions in different situations.

v) Emotions influence the psychological climate

In the home, school, neighbourhood and playgroup child's emotional expressions affect the psychological climate of his environment.

vi) Emotions influence physical growth

The positive and negative emotional expressions like love or the lack of it, good or poor discipline, bitter or sweet family relationship will all determine the rate and pattern of his physical and personality growth.

IV. Mental Development

Mental development is also a part of cognitive development. As the child develops, he makes increasingly complex adaptive responses to his physical and social environment. A one year old child is far superior in ability as compared with his capacity at birth. Individual differences are seen in the mental ability of children.

Factors affecting Mental development

i) Pre-natal Conditions

Illness and stress during pregnancy affect the mental level of the child.

ii) Social Class

A greater percentage of the very bright children come from families of superior socio-economic classes where the number of backward children is proportionally greater among the families of lower socio economic status. The parents from superior society have a high educational level. They live in healthy environment in superior residential areas. They have better chances of reading books and other reading materials. The development of intelligence is highly influenced by the richness of the learning opportunities. Large families sometimes can provide a learning environment but poor opportunities for continuing education than small families.

iii) Sex

It is seen that boys at all ages generally outrank girls in general information specially along scientific lines. The intelligence level of girls is high in linguistic and perceptual skills and in certain types of memories whereas boys have better insight into mathematical and engineering relationship.

iv) Nutrition

Malnutrition is caused by deficits of proper nutrients, diet and supplement needed for normal growth and development. During the months before birth and through the early childhood years, malnutrition influences cognitive development. It affects child's memory and ability to learn. Malnutrition may also cause different diseases such as diarrhea. A malnourished child cannot make enough enzymes to digest his food normally. This food which he cannot digest and absorb goes out of him/her in the form of stools.

v) Stimulation

A dull unhygienic environment also retards mental development of a child. When the child goes to school he normally makes up the lack of stimulation, but that is not sufficient to develop the skill and ability with which the child was born.

V. Language Development

The possession of ability to speak is one of the most distinguishing features which keep man apart from the animals. Speech also forms a relationship between language and thought. The word of the language has a wide variety of meanings; the forms of language are also different – it may be written, spoken or shown by way of sign and gestures.

Language is a primary means of social intercourse used not only to share people's own feelings or to express their own views but also to awaken a response in other people and to influence their attitudes and behaviour. The expression of mental content including both ideas and feelings through language considers that communication is a secondary function of language.

Language is closely associated with learning and memory. Language develops along with other development in the child including postural control, feeding behaviour and dentition. A very young child learns to differentiate his/her mother's voice and also learns to understand the meaning of crossness in her voice.

Language also improves as children mature. The child works out rules for speech as he hears. Language also develops through social contacts. The infant's language does not consist simply of babbling but it also reveals some efforts to imitate language spoken around him/her. At first stage of childhood, it is completely an imitative process.

Factors Affecting Language Development

i) Intelligence

The intellectually gifted child usually speaks earlier and more efficiently, while the mentally retarded child speaks later and articulates poorly. Children of high IQ show marked superiority both in size of vocabulary and in length and correctness of sentences structure.

ii) Hearing

It seems probable that infants think before they talk, but once they talk, speech influences their thought. The thought processes are similar in normal and deaf children.

iii) Health

Severe and prolonged illness during the first two years of life delays the beginning of speech and the use of sentences. All the needs of the sick child are fulfilled by the people around him.

iv) Maturation

Maturation plays a vital role in language development. Babbling which begins at about 7 months coincides approximately with standing up and the first real word comes with standing.

v) Sex

Apparently language functions develop earlier in girls than in boys. At every stage boys make less grammatic and shorter sentences than girls. The difference becomes more prominent with every passing year.

vi) Family Relationship

Language development is also dependent on family relationships because the child must have sufficient communication with more mature speakers to obtain information. Generally the mother is child's first language teacher. The father's role in children's language development is also very important.

vii) Size of Family

Size of the family also influences the child's language development. The only child for example gets a greater deal of parental attention and does not have any sibling rivalry.

VI. Social Development

Children grow socially as they grow physically from year to year, developing greater self-control, greater complexity of skills and social behaviour in getting along with people. Group relationships are important both for the individual and society. Learning to be a social person does not occur overnight. The child learns in cycles. Social development is an orderly process in each child.

A social child is one who behaves in a socially approved manner, plays the role which society prescribes for him and has favourable attitudes towards people and social activities. The child will be approved socially if he fits into the group and is accepted as a group member. Social development means acquisition of the ability to behave in accordance with social customs and expectations.

Factors Affecting Social Development

i) Ordinal Position

The position of the child in the family also affects social development. The elder, middle and the youngest child all will have different intensities for social development. The only child is often less social. Children with sibling of the same sex find it difficult to associate with other children of the opposite sex. The most favoured position is the second or younger of two children.

ii) Family Relationship

From infancy, family relationship is important for social development. Infants who have more physical and verbal contact with their mothers and with other persons around them show more interactions both with the mother and with strangers than children with fewer interpersonal contacts. Parents who assign responsibilities to the children help in encouraging the cooperative attitude among children. Children are forced to incline affection and approval elsewhere when their parents show active or passive neglect to them.

iii) Size of the Family

The size of the family in which the child grows up not only influences his/her early social experiences but also develops his/her social attitudes and pattern of behaviour. An only child gets more attention which is good for him.

iv) Parental Expectations

Parental expectations motivate the children's efforts to be socially recognized. The children normally learn to be polite and chivalrous to win love from their parents and other persons around them.

v) Teachers

The role of teachers is also very important for developing child's social adjustment.

They can help to make a child social and friendly by directing them in a right way. The teacher is often a role model to the young children. Even though the child is in school for only five or six hours a day, a teacher who is explosive, irritable and nagging may create many emotional reverberations. The child will need a very friendly home atmosphere to balance such a school situation.

Routine Habits and Personal Cleanliness of Children

The proper management of following sanitation routine affects the general health of children and keeps them away from many diseases.

i) Elimination

The elimination of waste products is necessary for the well being of the whole body. Children should be habituated with a regular time for this. Other routine habits include feeding, bathing, going to bed etc, regulate this habit.

ii) Urine control

This is one of the important routine habits of children which needs to be regulated. The children between 1.5 to 2 years should be taught not to wet their own clothes or pass urine anywhere except laratories.

iii) Brushing teeth

Massaging gum or brushing teeth with a finger or with a brush should be taught to the child as early as possible. He should learn to clean his teeth regularly in the morning and after every meal to avoid dental cavities. Sugar normally deposits on teeth and after fermentation dental cavities are developed. The worst delinquents are sweets, candies, chocolates, toffees or anything sugary that sticks to the teeth. To avoid such a problem, children should be encouraged to wash their mouth.

iv) Regular bathing

Bathing regularly is also considered to be another important habit to keep children healthy and free from many diseases which may develop in a dirty body. A warm or cold bath should be given to children everyday. Messaging oil before a bath is good for the skin of children. The daily bath increases the blood circulation in blood capillaries. The cleaning of hair is also very important to avoid dandruff and ticks in them.

v) Cleaning nails

Many unwanted substances are deposited in nails which are harmful for the health of children. Dirty nails may many fungal infections. The children should be taught to keep their nails clean. The cutting of the nails at regular intervals is also necessary.

vi) Clothing

Clothing should be selected according to the season. The clothes which are in direct contact with the body should normally be cotton, since cotton helps in the absorption of sweat. Woolen clothes help in preserving bodily heat. In winter if proper woolen clothes are not used and heat is lost, then to secure against heat loss children have to eat more heat-giving foodstuffs. Terylene and nylon are more durable and easily washable clothes but they catch fire easily. Cleanliness of clothes is also as important as personal (bodily) cleanliness. Dirty clothes may produce bad odour and may cause many skin diseases in children.

Play

Play is a spontaneous activity. It is the first work that child learns to do. Through play, children train themselves for useful work when they grow up. Play also helps to build a healthy physique and a beautiful mind. It is also essential for the development of a normal, well adjusted personality. Play has many values for young children. The most important are:

i) Outlet for extra energy.

ii) Development of all parts of the body-bones, muscles and internal organs.

iii) It is an exercise which develops good appetite and healthy sleep.

iv) Play enables the child to learn how to control the body.

v) Play develops many skills that will be useful all through his life.

vi) Encouragement of creativity.

vii) Development of the ability to keep the mind on the task at hand.

viii) Play is the best way to get rid of many emotional outbursts like anger, fear, jealousy and grief.

Children suffering from many frustrations, emotional deprivations and lack of understanding on the part of his parents can be treated with play therapy. It reduces psychic tension and helps the child to accept himself as he is with all his limitations.

Estimates of the destitute children in Developing Countries

A number of studies have shown that there is a keen relationship between poverty and cognitive development of children. Large gaps between richest and poorest children in school enrolment, early dropout, scores attained and achievements are particularly found in Sub Saharan Africa and South Asia. In Zambia, poor children enroll at the primary level four times later than the rich children. In Uganda, the problem is more severe. In Jamaica, 74% of total 5000 children from rich families have entered in the fee paying nursery schools while 41% of 25000 children have enrolled in the free government aided primary schools. In Punjab (India), figures shown by Department of Education (2007) do not give a very positive picture of the infrastructure facilities available in the schools of Punjab. There are 676 schools at the primary level without their main building. 78 per cent require more toilets, 39 per cent require boundary walls, 30 per cent verandas and 49 per cent require usable play ground. Drinking water, which is a basic necessity is also not available in 20 per cent of the schools. Further information and data collected from the Directorate of Education too indicates that many of these buildings are in a dilapidated condition and have been declared unsafe for use as classrooms.

Conclusion and Policy Implications

Welfare and income support policies are based on economic thinking whereas many child policies are rooted in child development, early child education and related fields.

Welfare and income support policies are designed to influence parents' employment (especially maternal employment), income and material resources and family structure are likely in turn to influence children's family environment, community environment, physical and material environment. Environmental contexts that support a decent quality of life can be justified on that basis alone, but they are also important because they can affect children's physical, intellectual and socio-emotional development.

Low income children who experience unstable child care, frequent changes and multiple arrangements tend to have more behavioural problems in them than those with more stable child care. Changing child care arrangements may be a sign of instability in other facets of family life. Three key strategies address what is most important for low-income children: i) helping families to achieve an adequate standard of living ii) helping them to provide stable and supportive homes and iii) helping them to access quality child care.

A family's economic resources influence child well-being because they are necessary to meet children's basic needs for food and shelter.

In India, the Central government, in partnership with state governments, has initiated a number of programmes to fulfill the constitutional responsibilities and national objectives. Under this joint scheme, free and compulsory primary education would be provided. Mid–day Meal has been continuing since 1995. Free text books to all the female students and the entire scheduled castes and scheduled tribes students up to the primary level have been provided under "Sarv Shiksha Abhiyan" (SSA) scheme. At present every state is hopeful of achieving universalization of primary education within a decade through this scheme. The major thrusts in SSA are as follows:

i) All 6-14 age group children have to enroll in school by 2010.

ii) All 6-14 age group children have to complete five years of schooling by 2012.

iii) All 6-14 age group children have to complete eight years of schooling by 2015.

(Anusri Mallik is currently working as a Faculty Associate in Icfai Research Centre, Kolkata. The author can be reached at anusri.mallik@gmail.com).

References

1. Basu, K., P. H. Van (1998). "The Economics of Child Labor", The American Economic Review, 88(3), pp. 412-427.
2. Behrman, J. R., M. R. Rosenzweig (2002), "Does Increasing Women's Schooling Raise the Schooling of the Next Generation?", The American Economic Review, Vol. 92, No. 1., pp. 323- 334.
3. Bradley R, Corwyn R. Socioeconomic status and child development. Ann Rev Psychol 2002; 53: 371–99.
4. Bredy T, Humpartzoomian R, Cain D, Meaney M. Partial reversal of the effect of maternal care on cognitive function through environmental enrichment. Neurosci 2003; 118: 571–6.
5. Brooks-Gunn J, Duncan GJ. The effects of poverty on children. Future Child 1997; 7: 55–71.
6. Cigno, A. (2006), "A Constitutional Theory of the Family", Journal of Population Economics, 19, pp. 259–283.
7. Cigno, A., F.C. Rosati (2000), "Mutual Interest, Self-enforcing Constitutions and Apparent Generosity". In L. A. Ge´rard-Varet, S. C. Kolm, J. M. Ythier (Eds.), The Economics of Reciprocity, Giving and Altruism. London and New York: MacMillan and St Martin's Press. 24
8. Cochrane, S.H., D.K. Guilkey (1995), "The Effects of Fertility Intentions and Access to Services on Contraceptive Use in Tunisia". Economic Development and Cultural Change, 43, pp. 779-804.
9. Degraff, D.S., R.E. Bilsborrow, D.K. Guilkey (1997), "Community-Level Determinants of Contraceptive Use in the Philippines: A Structural Analysis". Demography, 34, pp. 385-398.
10. Desai, S., D. Jain (1994), "Maternal Employment and Changes in Family Dynamics: the Social Context of Women's Work in Rural India", Population and Development Review, 115-136.

11 Francavilla, F., G.C. Giannelli G. C. (2007), "The Relation between Child Labour and Mother's Work: the case of India" IZA DP 3099, Bonn. Giannelli, G.C., F.

12. Francavilla (2007), "Do family Planning Programmes Help Womens' Employment? The Case of Indian Mothers", IZA DP 2762, Bonn.

13. IIPS, International Institute for Population Sciences, ORC Macro (2000). "National Family Health Survey (NFHS-2)", 1998–99 India. Mumbai: IIPS.

14. Plug, E. (2004), "Estimating the Effect of Mother's Schooling on Children's Schooling Using a Sample of Adoptees", The American Economic Review, Vol. 94, No. 1., pp. 358-368.

15. Rutstein, S.H., K. Johnson (2004), "DHS Comparative Reports. The DHS Wealth Index", No. 6, ORC Macro Calverton, Maryland USA.

16. Rabe-Hesketh, S., A. Skrondal, , A. Pickles (2004), "Gllamm manual". U.C. Berkeley Division of Biostatistics, Working Paper Series 160.

17. Rosenzweig MR, Wolpin KI. Are there increasing returns to the intergenerational production of human capital—maternal schooling and child intellectual achievement. J Hum Res 1994; 29: 670–93.

18. Skrondal, A., S. Rabe-Hesketh (2004), Generalised Latent Variable Modelling. CRC/ Chapman Hall.

19. Yeung, J., F.W. Sandberg, P. E. Davis-Kean, S.L. Hofferth (2001), "Children's Time with Fathers in Intact Families", Journal of Marriage and the Family, Vol. 63, No. 1., pp. 136-154.

20. UNICEF, (2007), The State of the World's Children. Women and Children, UN New York.

21. UNICEF, (2008), The State of the World's Children. Child Survival, UN New York.

22. Victora CG, Wagstaff A, Schellenberg JA, Gwatkin D, Claeson M, Habicht JP. Applying an equity lens to child health and mortality: more of the same is not enough. Lancet 2003; 362: 233–41.

23. Wooldridge, J.M. (2002), Econometric Analysis of Cross Section and Panel Data, MIT Press, Cambridge, MA. 25.

2

What Matter for Child Development?

Fali Huang

This paper estimates production functions of child cognitive and social development using a panel data of nine-year old children each with over two hundred home and school inputs as well as family background variables. A tree regression method is used to conduct estimation under various specifications. A small subset of inputs is found consistently important in explaining variances of child development results, including the number of books a child has at various ages and how often a mother reads to child by age five, while the effects of race and maternal employment are negligible when detailed inputs are controlled.

1. Introduction

An old Chinese saying claims that a person's lifetime achievements can be well predicted by his performance at age seven. Its validity in modern times is confirmed by recent evidence. In Britain, for example, a person's test scores at age seven are significantly associated with his education level and earnings in thirties (Currie and Thomas 2001). In the US, skill endowment heterogeneity at age sixteen may account for ninety percent of the total variance of individual lifetime earnings

(Keane and Wolpin 1997). One possible reason for the vital importance of skill formation in early childhood is that success or failure at this stage leads to success or failure in school which in turn leads to success or failure in post-school learning (Heckman 1999).

The main goal of this paper is to estimate production functions of early child cognitive and social development results. Since home and school inputs are often endogenous choices of parents and hence are correlated with each other and across periods, any omitted inputs would necessarily cause bias in estimated effects of included ones. To minimize the omitted variable problem, this paper adopts various within-child difference and value-added specifications to deal with the unobserved family and child fixed factors, and uses a comprehensive set of detailed inputs: Based on National Longitudinal Surveys 1979 Youth (NLSY79) data in the US, we construct a sample of 4726 eight and nine-year-old children with over two hundred inputs from mother's prenatal care until current period.[1]

Current scientific knowledge, however, does not tell us which inputs among the two hundred plus available ones in the data affect child development and how they may interact with each other. Furthermore, most inputs are measured by categorical variables with multiple items, and many contain missing values. Researchers faced with these problems are often forced to choose, quite arbitrarily, which variables to include in and what structures to impose on production functions, how to combine different categories, and how to handle missing variables. Important information may be lost during this subjective data reduction process (Harvey 1999), and different treatments *per se* may give rise to discrepant estimation results even for the same data (Haveman and Wolfe 1995). This motivates us to adopt a non-parametric method, namely tree structured regression, in estimation. The optimization mechanism underlying the tree regression is similar to the conventional linear regression; its non-parametric features are designed to select important explanation variables, detect non-linear structures, and treat missing values in a systematic way (Breiman, Friedman, Olshen, and Stone 1984).[2]

The estimation results in various specifications yield a consistent picture, where a reasonably small set of earlier and current inputs are important predictors for child development results at age eight or nine. The number of books a child has at various ages and how often a mother reads to her child before age 5 are the most important predictors of child math and reading scores from age five onwards; they are also primary predictors of child behavior problem scores at age 5. Spanking a child aged 8-9 seems to be mostly driven by family or child fixed factors and have no effects on current result, while spanking a younger child may reduce his future, behavior problems. When detailed home and school inputs are controlled, a mother's working hours in the first five years of a child's life have little effects on child development results at age 8-9; so does a child s race or sex.

There is a large body of literature studying the contributing factors to child cognitive and social-emotional development. A lot of work examines the effects of maternal employment on early child development results (Blau and Grossberg 1992, Parcel and Menahan 1994, Harvey 1999, Ruhm 2000, Waldfogel *et al.* 2002, Baum 2003). Most of these studies use linear regression models taking control of various family background variables. Their findings are mixed and no consensus has been reached, probably due to *ad hoc* selection of control variables and omitted variable problems mentioned above (Haveman and Wolfe 1995, Todd and Wolpin 2003). The current paper finds no effects of mother working on child development once detailed inputs are included. This is consistent with the finding of Waldfogel *et al.* (2002) that the effects of maternal employment are much reduced after a couple of home quality indicators are controlled. A possible explanation is that a mother's quality time with children is not much affected by her labor force participation (Bianchi 2000).

Another strand of literature examines the role of child care (e.g. NICHD ECCRN 2001, 2003). The overall quality of child care is found to be modestly related to child development outcomes, while family factors are more consistent predictors. This finding is also confirmed by our estimation results where the type of child care, the duration and intensity of child care experiences in the first three years never show up as primary explaining variables.

The paper shows that the racial gaps of math and reading scores among eight and nine year-old children can be completely accounted for by home and school inputs. This is a striking result since a substantial Black-White test score gap persists even after controlling for a wide range of characteristics (Fryer and Levitt 2004, Todd and Wolpin 2004).

The school inputs in general have less explanation power than home inputs. This is consistent with the finding of Parcel and Durfur (2001) that the effects of school inputs on child behavior are modest in size, while home inputs are stronger. Similarly, the standard school inputs such as class size, pupil-teacher ratio, and teacher experiences are usually found to have little effect on children attainment (Feinstein and Symons 1999).

The results also suggest that, though earlier scores are very important in predicting future results, they may not be sufficient statistics for historical inputs. Indeed, some earlier inputs have direct effects on current child performance beyond what is already captured by earlier scores. For example, the number of books a child has at age seven and how often his mother reads to him around age three are primary indicators of his math and reading scores at age nine, even when corresponding scores at age seven are controlled.

The paper is organized as follows. The childhood history sample is described in section 2. Regression tree analysis and various estimation methods are discussed in the subsequent two sections. The results of regression trees are presented in section 5. The final section concludes.

2. Data: Childhood History Samples

Starting from 1986, children born to mothers included in National Longitudinal Surveys 1979 Youth (NLSY79) are surveyed every two years. The set of child development results and inputs from birth up to 10 years is different across three age-groups, namely 0-2 years, 3-5 years, and 6-9 years. We construct a sample of 4726 children each of whom has a single pair of comparable scores and inputs at ages 6-7 and 8-9, plus historical inputs at ages 0-5, mother's prenatal care, mother's working history up to the fifth year after child birth, and family backgrounds. For children five years old and above, the cognitive development is measured by PIAT (Peabody Individual Achievement Test) math and reading recognition scores, while social and behavioral development is measured by BPI (Behavior Problem Index) Total Scores.

A brief introduction of home and school inputs as well as maternal working and family backgrounds is in order. For children age three and above, home environment variables include how many books a child has, how often a mother reads to child, how often a father plays with him outdoors, whether there are musical instruments and newspapers at home, whether parents encourage hobbies and bring a child to enriching activities, how often the family gets together with relatives and friends, how often a child watches TV and attends religious service etc. For younger children, home inputs also include the number of various toys a child has, how often he is talked to and taken to grocery shopping, whether he was breast-fed and how long the breast-feeding lasts, whether a mother teaches a child letters, numbers, and shapes, etc. The child care experiences in a child's first three years are measured by whether a child is in regular child care, the type of child care, the months per year and hours per week in child care. Variables about parenting styles include how often a child is expected to make bed, to clean room, etc., and how mother responds to low-grade tantrums, and hits. Mother's prenatal care variables include mother's usage of alcohol, cigarettes, vitamins, and sonograms during pregnancy, and whether a child has low birth weight. Maternal employment history covers a mother's working hours one year before child birth up to the fifth year afterwards. Family backgrounds include a mother's highest grades, AFQT scores, age at child birth, her marital status, her wages, the salary income and total family incomes, the region the family lives, whether the mother ever lived in her youth, whether there is a father figure at home, whether he is the biological father, etc. The school inputs include school types, number of hours a child works on homework, mother's rating of school quality including teacher skill and caring of students, safety of school, moral teaching, etc.

3. Regression Tree Analysis

A regression tree is a piecewise linear estimate of a regression function constructed by recursively partitioning the data.[3] It is grown by sequentially splitting the sample into binary nodes/subsets. At each node, every explaining variable competes in its ability to reduce the node variance; the variable with the best improvement score is selected to be the *primary splitter.* Unlike the linear regression, here not all available predictors show up as primary splitters: The primary splitters must be the best predictive variable at some node. The tree growing process continues until the variances in all nodes are less than some threshold. The tree is then pruned backwards to get a sequence of trees with different number of terminal nodes; the pruning rule balances the trade-off between the out-of-sample resubstitution errors and the complexity of the trees. From this whole sequence the *optimal tree* is selected using test sample or cross-validation error estimate.[4] The *importance* of a variable measures its overall ability as a primary splitter in an optimal tree to explain the variance of dependent variable in all nodes; it corresponds to the variable's total effect on the dependent variable.

Overall, the accuracy of regression tree has been generally competitive with linear regression. It can be much more accurate on non-linear problems, though it tends to be somewhat less accurate on problems with good linear structure; this is not a problem here since most variables are categorical. A main drawback of the tree regression, determined by its non-parametric characteristics, is that it does not provide the traditional statistical significant tests. However, variables selected as primary splitters tend to be also significant in the conventional sense since they are the best predictive variables among many available ones and their predictive abilities are further tested on a random test sample.[5]

4. Estimation Methods

We run tree regressions according to various specifications used in the literature. The simplest estimation method uses only contemporaneous home and school inputs, labeled *current input regression*, which yields unbiased estimates when only current inputs matter and when they are unrelated to unobserved child ability. The *historical input regression* includes both current and historical inputs; if some historical inputs act as primary splitters, then current input regressions are biased.

One way to allow for unobserved child ability is using an earlier score as its proxy. The *value-added historical regression* includes an earlier score in addition to current and historical inputs. If historical inputs act as primary splitters, it suggests they have direct effects on future child development and hence the earlier score is not a sufficient statistic for them.

Another way is to use *within-child difference regression*, where the regressant is the first difference in scores of the same child at different times, while regressors include both current and earlier inputs. This eliminates the effects of unobserved child ability and gets unbiased estimates when (1) child ability has the same effect on scores, (2) it does not interact with inputs in any non-linear way, and finally (3) input choices in the second period do not depend on the first period's random shock. The third condition can be explicitly checked since we have variables on how a mother responds to low grades and behavioral problems; it holds for cognitive development production functions but not so well for social and behavioral development. To further check the degree of endogeneity problem for disciplines, a regression is run using the behavior scores at age 7 as the dependent variable, while including future inputs at ages 8-9 as well as current and earlier inputs. Age 8-9 inputs would appear as primary splitters when the endogeneity problem is severe. But the opposite is true; actually the optimal regression tree does not change before and after including these future inputs. This evidence suggests the endogeneity problem is too weak to affect the main results.

5. Estimation Results

The main regression results are summarized in Tables 1-3, where the importance levels of primary splitters for the included regression trees are listed.[6] Recall that an input's importance measures its total effect on the dependent variable.

5.1 Math Scores for Children at Ages 8-9

Table 1 summarizes regression results for PIAT math scores. In the current input regression Current, race is the most important predictor. When it is excluded in 'C/race', however, the relative error increases by only 0.02, while the effects of books and TV watching hours at weekdays are almost doubled, and the degree of physical affection shown by mother to child as well as several other home inputs become primary splitters. When earlier inputs are included in 'History', the importance of race is halved compared with current. When race is excluded in 'H/race', many inputs become primary splitters including special activities and TV watching hours at weekdays, while the importance of existing primary splitters has little change. These results suggest that most effects of race on math scores can be accounted for by earlier and current inputs a child receives, though race is a good proxy for detailed home inputs when they are not available.

Comparing the two columns 'C/race' and 'H/race', it is clear that earlier inputs are important to PIAT math scores. In general, the importance of current inputs goes down in the historical input tree, which suggests that their estimated effects in current input tree are biased upward. For example, the importance of books at ages

8-9 is greatly reduced (from 15.3 to 1.29) while the number of books at ages 6-7 becomes the most important predictor.

In the value-added historical regression 'VAY' where PIAT math score at age 7 is used, earlier inputs such as books at ages 6-7 and mother reading to child at ages 3-5 still have positive effects, though their importance is reduced. This implies that the previous PIAT math score, though with very high importance, is not a sufficient statistic for earlier inputs. The only current input selected is a mother's physical affection for child.

The extreme importance of the math score at age 7 in predicting the score two years later may suggest that child's ability has large effects on math scores. But how does child's ability in math evolve over time? To shed some light on this question, the math score at age 5 is used as a proxy for child's ability in 'VAB'. The three primary splitters are the number of books at ages 6-7 and 8-9, and special activities at ages 8-9. The importance of math score at age 5 is much lower than that at age 7, while the total importance of inputs increases. One implication is that a child's ability in math is affected by home inputs especially books and enriching activities. The explaining power of inputs alone, however, is quite low since no optimal within-child tree exists for the math score.

Among all inputs, the number of books a child has at ages 6-7 and 8-9, mother's physical affection for child, special activities, and mother reading to child at ages 3-5 appear as primary splitters in at least one of the three value-added regressions.

5.2 Reading Scores for Children at Ages 8-9

Table 2 summarizes six regression trees for PIAT reading scores. For both current and historical input trees, regressions with and without race are strikingly similar. When historical inputs are included in column History, books at ages 6-7 becomes the most important input (with importance 18.7) and the importance of books at ages 8-9 is greatly reduced (from 19.8 to 3.52), which is exactly the same scenario as in the math score regressions. In the value-added historical tree VAY with reading score at ages 6-7, the top two inputs are books at age 7 and child's reading habit at ages 8-9. This implies that the earlier reading score is not a sufficient statistic for earlier inputs. In 'VAB' with ages 5 reading score, the aggregate importance of inputs is higher, which suggests the reading ability is also affected by home inputs. In within-child regression, the most important inputs are the number of books and child's reading habit at ages 8-9.

Overall, the number of books and a child's reading habit at ages 8-9 are the most important inputs predicting a child's reading scores at ages 8-9. The important inputs and their ranking are quite similar in both reading and math score regressions; a difference is that reading scores are affected by more inputs in value-added and within-child specifications.

5.3 Behavior Problem Scores for Children at Ages 8-9

Table 3 summarizes five BPI regression trees. The difference between current and historical input trees is quite small; the only earlier input that matters is spanking frequency at ages 6-7, while the importance levels of spanking and grounding a child at ages 8-9 do not change. In the value-added historical tree VAY using the BPI score at age 7, the frequencies of grounding and sending a child to room are still primary splitters, though the importance of grounding is much reduced; in contrast, the large effect of spanking at ages 8-9 disappears. Since no earlier inputs show up, the age 7 BPI score seems to be a sufficient statistic for both ability and earlier inputs.

When the BPI score at age 5 is used in VAB, the number of grounding and room-sending at ages 8-9 are still the most important inputs. Many other inputs also become primary splitters including some inputs at ages 3-5, so BPI score at age 5 is not a sufficient statistic for earlier inputs. The relative error in VAB is only 0.015 points higher than VAY, which suggests the difference between BPI scores at ages 5 and 7 can be mostly accounted for by home inputs. The within-child tree using age 5 BPI score is presented in the last column, where spanking a child at ages 3 5 is negatively (though modestly) associated with his behavior problem at ages 8-9, while the opposite is true for sending a child to room at ages 8-9. The errors are very high, and now within-child tree exists using ages 7 BPI score.

In these behavior problem regressions, the number of times sending a child to room, grounding him, and how often he reads for self-enjoyment at ages 8-9 are selected as primary splitters in most specifications even when an earlier score is controlled. In sharp contrast, though the current spanking frequency is the most important predictor in both current and historical input trees, it never appears in any value-added or within-child difference specifications. This suggests spanking a child of ages 8-9 merely reflects some family- or child-specific fixed factors. Spanking a child at ages 3-5, however, is negatively associated with his behavior problem at ages 8-9 as shown in the within-child regression.

5.4 Child Development Results at Age 5

A common feature of the various regressions above is that child development results at age 5 are very important for future outcomes. So it is interesting to know how the age 5 results are affected by home inputs. The results are briefly described below, though the detailed table is omitted. The number of books and how often a mother reads to child at ages 3-5 are important for both cognitive and social development, while the latter is the most important input for math and reading scores; the spanking frequency at ages 3-5 is the best predictor of BPI scores at age 5. Race matters only for math score, and again its effect is partially accounted for by books, reading to child, and birth order.

Overall, books and how often a mother reads to her child appear to matter most for child's cognitive development at age 5; they are also the primary predictors for behavior problems at age 5, though spanking is most predictive. The errors are generally higher than corresponding regressions of child development results at ages 8-9.

6. Conclusion

Early child development is a crucial part of human capital formation. The paper estimates production functions of child's cognitive and social development at ages 8-9 using NLSY(79) child data, where over two hundred home- and school-inputs starting from mother's prenatal care periods are included as well as many family background variables. A tree structured regression method is used to conduct estimation, and the unobserved family or child heterogeneity is handled by within-child difference and value-added specifications. The omitted variable problem is greatly mitigated by using a very rich set of detailed inputs and further checked by including family backgrounds in the regressions. The endogeneity problem of disciplinary inputs is checked by putting future inputs at ages 8-9 into the regressions of child development results at age 7. The evidence shows that the influence of this problem, if any, is very weak.

Detailed home inputs are found to be the most important predictors of child development results. Production functions of child's math and reading scores are more similar to each other than to behavior problem scores. The number of books a child has at various ages, how often a child reads for self-enjoyment, and how often a mother reads to her child before age 5 are among the most important inputs predicting math and reading scores from age 5 onwards. A child's behavior problem score at ages 8-9 is mostly correlated with parental disciplining such as how often he gets grounded or sent to room, while the score at age 5 is also affected by how often his mother reads to him and the number of books he had. Spanking a child aged 8-9 has no effects on current results, while spanking a younger child may reduce his future behavior problems.

A reasonably small set of inputs from over two hundred available in the data are selected as primary predictors for child cognitive and social development results at age 8 and 9, which may be used as a rough guide for variable selection in relevant research. Though there is some evidence suggesting the estimated effects of these home and school inputs are more than correlations, future research is needed to further establish the causal links.

(Fali Huang, School of Economics and Social Sciences, Singapore Management University.)

Endnotes

1 Even with this rich data set, one may still worry about omitted variable problems. To check this, we include in the regressions many family background variables, which should be correlated with omitted inputs. Since they never show up as primary explaining predictors, it suggests that the influence of omitted variables, if any, is very modest.

2 This is the first time regression tree analysis is used extensively in child development area, though it has been applied in medical, biological, weather forecasting and many other areas. In economics and finance literature, it was used occasionally to detect regime shifting patterns (e.g. Durlauf and Johnson, 1995).

3 There are various ways in conducting tree regressions. The one used here, also the mostly widely used, is CART (Classification And Regression Tree) established by Breiman *et al.* (1984). The tree regression can be conducted in a similar manner as implementing linear regressions using a standard statistical software.

4 Take the test sample estimate as an example. A subset is selected randomly from the whole sample as the *learning sample* to grow the mother tree, while the remaining one is the independent *test sample*. Use each subtree on the test sample to predict the dependent variable and calculate the resulted sum of squared errors; the subtree with the minimum relative test error (compared to mean squared error) is selected as the optimal tree.

5 Though it is technically not feasible to replicate the tree analysis using linear regression for the current project, I did try to use the linear regression method by reducing the categorical variables to binary versions, ignoring any interactive terms, and omitting missing values. The main results are similar: the family background and child care variables are rarely significant, while the home inputs selected as primary explaining variables in the tree regressions are often significant in the OLS as well.

6 Detailed regression trees are available upon request.

References

[1] Baum, C.L., 2003, Does Early Maternal Employment Harm Child Development? An Analysis of the Potential Bene ts of Leave-Taking, Journal of Labor Economics 21(2), 409-448.

[2] Bianchi, S.M., 2000, Maternal Employment and Time with Children: Dramatic Change or Surprising Continuity?, Demography 37(4), 401-414.

[3] Blau, F.D. and A.J. Grossberg, 1992, Maternal Labor Supply and Children's Cognitive Development, The Review of Economics And Statistics, 474-481.

[4] Breiman, L., J. Friedman, R. Olshen, and C.J. Stone, 1984, Classification and Regression Trees, Chapman and Hall, New York.

[5] Currie, J. and D. Thomas, 2001, Early Test Scores, Socioeconomic Status, School Quality and Future Outcomes, Research in Labor Economics 20, 103-132.

[6] Durlauf, S.N. and P.A. Johnson, 1995, Multiple Regimes and Cross-Country Growth Behavior, Journal of Applied Econometrics 10, 365-384.

[7] Feinstein, L. and J. Symons, 1999, Attainment in Secondary School, Oxford Economic Papers 51, 300-321.

[8] Fryer, R.G. Jr. and S. Levitt, 2004, Understanding the Black-White Test Score Gap in the First Two Years of School, Review of Economics and Statistics 86(2), 447-464.

[9] Hastie, T., R. Tibshirani, and J. Friedman, 2001, The Elements of Statistical Learning: Data mining, Inference, and Prediction, New York: Springer.

[10] Harvey, E., 1999, Short-Term and Long-Term Effects of Early Parental Employment on Children of the NLSY, Developmental Psychology 35(2), 445-459.

[11] Haverman, R. and B. Wolfe, 1995, The Determinants of Children's Attainments: A Review of Methods and Findings, Journal of Economic Literature XXXIII, 1829-78.

[12] Heckman, J., 1999, Policies to Foster Human Capital, NBER working paper #7288.

[13] NICHD ECCRN (Early Child Care Research Network), 2001, Nonmaternal care and family factors in early development: An overview of the NICHD Study of Early Child Care, Journal of Applied Developmental Psychology 22, 457-492.

[14] NICHD ECCRN, 2003, Does amount of time spent in child care predict socioemotional adjustment during the transition to kindergarten?, Child Development 74, 976-1005.

[15] Parcel, T.L. and E.G. Menaghan, 1994, Early Parental Work, Family Social Capital, and Early Childhood Outcomes, American Journal of Sociology 99(4), 972-1009.

[16] Parcel, T. L. and M.J. Dufur, 2001, Capital at Home and at School: Effects on Child Social Adjustment, Journal of Marriage and the Family 63(1), 32-47.

[17] Ruhm, C.J., 2000, Parental Employment and Child Cognitive Development, Journal of Human Resources 19(6), 931-960.

[18] Todd, P.E. and K.I. Wolpin, 2003, Towards a Unified Approach for Modeling the Production Function for Cognitive Achievement, Economic Journal, F3-F33.

[19] Todd, P.E. and K.I. Wolpin, 2004, The Production of Cognitive Achievement in Children: Home, School and Racial Test Score Gaps, working paper, University of Pennsylvania.

[20] Waldfogel, J., W. Han, and J. Brooks-Gunn, 2002, The Effects of Early Maternal Employment on Child Cognitive Development, Demography 39(2), 369-392.

Table 1: Effects of Home and School Inputs on PIAT Math Scores at Age 8-9

Inputs	Current	C/race	History	H/race	VAY	VAB
Current inputs at age 8-9						
# of books a child has	6.04	15.3	1.29	1.29		2.53
# of hours/weekday child sees TV	3.07	6.07		2.82		
# showing child physical affection	3.12		0.75	1.02		
How often child reads for enjoyment	2.39	2.62	2.79	2.48		
Child gets special help w/remedial work	3.42	1.98		1.10		
# past week mom spanked child	1.46	1.24	1.66			
Child gets special lessons/activities	1.39			4.46		2.74
Mom keeps closer eye if low grades		1.09	0.96			
Mom responds to tantrum-time out	1.48					
Mom responds to tantrum-talk with child	1.24	1.23				
parents participate with school	1.22					
Earlier inputs						
# of books a child has at age 6-7	–	–	17.4	17.4	1.40	2.14
teacher caring of child at age 6-7	–	–		1.26		
# of books a child has at age 3-5	–	–	1.91	1.45		
Mom helps child learn shapes at age 3-5	–	–	1.71	1.91		
Child has record/tape player at age 3-5	–	–	1.27			
How often mother reads to child at age 3-5	–	–	1.05		0.59	
Race (White versus Black/Hispanic)	15.95	–	7.72	–		
Earlier Scores						
PIAT math score at age 7	–	–	–	–	67.7	–
PIAT math score at age 5	–	–	–	–	–	39.8
Sample Variance	190	190	190	190	190	194
Sum of Squared Errors on test sample	0.83	0.85	0.844	0.838	0.65	0.79
Sample Size	2992	2992	2992	2992	2992	2008

Notes: The entries are the importance levels of inputs, which measures its total effect on the dependent variable. Current—Only current inputs at ages 8-9 included; C/race if race excluded. History—Historical inputs included; H/race if race excluded. VAY—Value-added regression with age 7 score and all inputs. VAB—Value-added regression with age 5 score and all Inputs. Some inputs with importance less than one are not listed in the table. In the 'C/race' they are: how often mom reads to child, how often child eats w/parents, is there music instrument at home, and # times mom says positive things in past week. In the 'H/race' they are: how often child taken to performance, whether child gets special assignment for advanced work, limits non-school activity if low grades, # mom grounded child in past week, how often child is expected to bathe self, child ever sees father-figure at ages 6-7, birth order, # child reads for enjoyment at ages 6-7, mom responds to hit-send to room at age 3-5, hours mom worked/week 4th quarter and 5th year after child birth, and how often child eats with parents by age 2.

Table 2: Effects of Home and School Inputs on PIAT Reading Scores of at Age 8-9

Inputs	Current	C/race	History	VAY	Within	VAB
Current inputs at age 8-9						
# of books a child has	19.8	19.8	3.52		2.99	3.18
How often child reads for enjoyment	8.9	8.9	9.28	2.51	2.37	
Child gets special help w/remedial work	10.3	10.3	10.7			3.97
How often child eats with parents	1.67	1.67				0.6
#times past week mom spanked child	1.60	1.60		1.59		
Parents participate with school	1.40					
Child gets special lessons/activities	1.21	2.40				
How often child w/ dad outdoors					1.01	
Mom rating of teacher caring					0.92	
Mom punishes child for low grades					0.68	
School communicates with parents		1.15				
# hours/weekend day child sees TV		1.08				
How often child expected to clean room						1.34
Earlier inputs						
# of books a child has at ages 6-7	–		18.7	3.57		3.91
# past week child spanked at ages 6-7	–				1.66	
# mom shows child affection at ages 6-7	–				0.68	
# child reads for enjoyment at ages 6-7	–				1.95	
# past week child grounded at ages 6-7	–				1.59	
Child has record/tape player at ages 3-5	–		2.7			
Mom's attitude on child learning by age 3	–		1.55			
How often mother reads to child by age 3	–				0.70	
Race (White vs. Black/Hispanic)	2.68	–	2.13		0.96	
Earlier scores						
PIAT reading score at age 7	–	–	–	97.8	–	–
PIAT reading score at age 5	–	–	–	–	–	55
Sample Variance	221	221	221	221	120	224
Sum of Squared Errors on test sample	0.825	0.827	0.835	0.57	0.966	0.74
Sample Size	2982	2982	2982	2982	2982	1935

Notes: The entries are the importance levels of inputs, which measures its total effect on the dependent variable. Current—Only current inputs at ages 8-9 included; C/race if race excluded. History—Historical inputs included; H/race if race excluded. VAY—Value-added regression with age 7 score and all inputs. VAB—Value-added regression with age 5 score and all Inputs. Within —Within-child regression using age 7 score and all inputs.

Table 3: Effects of Home and School Inputs on BPI Total Scores at Age 8-9

Inputs	**Current**	**History**	**VAY**	**VAB**	**Within**
#times past week mom spanked child	19.6	19.6			
#times past week mom grounded child	9.9	9.9	3.11	8.24	
#times past week mom sent child to room	4.65	4.0	3.98	4.14	3.92
How often child reads for enjoyment	3.93	1.84		1.09	1.53
How often family gets with relatives and friends	2.45				
How often child picks up after self				1.27	
Mom sees if child improves on own for low grades				0.92	
#times past week mom said positive things				0.61	
Earlier inputs					
# times past week mom spanked child at ages 6-7	–	4.49		1.67	
# times past week mom took away TV at ages 6-7	–				1.81
How often child w/ dad outdoors at ages 6-7	–			1.35	
#times past week mom spanked child at ages 3-5	–				1.31
Mom responds to hit-send to room at ages 3-5	–			1.05	
Mom helps child learn alphabets at ages 3-5	–			0.96	
Earlier scores BPI total score at age 7	–	–	79.6	–	–
BPI total score at age 5	–	–	–	51	–
Sample Variance	221	221	221	221	195
Sum of Squared Errors on test sample	0.87	0.86	0.68	0.69	0.98
Sample Size	3021	3021	3021	3021	2512

Notes: The entries are the importance levels of inputs, which measures its total effect on the dependent variable. Current—Only current inputs at ages 8-9 included. History—Historical inputs included. VAY—Value-added regression with age 7 score and all inputs. VAB—Value-added regression with age 5 score and all Inputs. Within—Within-child regression using age 5 score and all inputs.

3

Child Health: Concepts and Issues

Dalia Dey and Kasturi Nandy

"Tomorrow's world is already taking shape in the body and spirit of children."

The Millennium Development Goal 4, aims to reduce child mortality rate by two-thirds, by 2015. The global scenario needs much attention, to achieve this target. This article focuses on different measures of child health, in terms of infant mortality rate, immunization rate, child malnutrition, etc. According to the authors, race, gender, poverty, industrialization, are a few factors which are affecting the health of a child. The article also throws some light on the interventions made by the government and other non-governmental organizations with an aim to improve child health.

Introduction

Health is an index of human welfare and is a major contributing factor to the economic growth of a nation. It is considered to be an asset which enables a person to develop his potential, which in turn, increases the productivity of a person individually as well as to a whole nation. A healthy body leads to a healthy mind which positively increases productivity. According to the Nobel Prize winner, Robert Fogel, health of

This article earlier published in the book "Child Health: Issues and Country Experiences" published by the Icfai University Press.

the people of a nation is linked to the economic growth of the nation. Children are the future of the nation. The health of today's children is the health of the future adults, which comprises the workforce. Health has a major effect on the strength of body and mind and the cognitive development of the child. A healthy and productive child can contribute to the workforce which adds value to the overall economic growth of a nation. The Millennium Development Goal (MDG) (Goal 4) aims to reduce child mortality rate among children under five by two thirds between 1990 to 2015. However, the poor countries have not been able to come close to the target set by MDG. The countries where the death rates are very high, are not yet getting adequate health care services.

Infant Mortality Rate (IMR) is the number of children dying before reaching one year of age, per 1000 live births. Child Mortality Rate (CMR) is the number of people dying before reaching age five, per 1000 live births. Dehydration, diarrhoea and pneumonia are some of the major causes risking the lives of infants. Besides, hygiene and sanitary conditions affect the child mortality and infant mortality rates. LDCs had seventeen times more IMR than the more developed countries.[1] Countries in Africa also have a high IMR. In fact, IMR has been found to increase in some of the countries in Sub-Saharan Africa. Lesser developed countries have a child mortality rate of 91 per 1000 live births whereas the condition in least developed nations is worse. The latter records child mortality rate of 161 out of 1000 live births[2]. Polio is another cause of disability which has led to about 1,939 cases of paralysis by January 2007.[3]

Present Status of Child Health: A Global Picture

In developing countries, in recent past, child mortality rate and the absolute number of annual deaths have declined substantially. Inspite of this fact, the shocking but true figures are – in developing nations nearly 11 million children (under 5 years) die in a year. About one million newborns do not survive beyond 24 hours. About 4 million are newborn among the total child deaths. The figures above are expressing the seriousness of this child mortality issue. About 10.5 million children who die every year, succumb to preventable diseases. The low and middle income countries are the worst affected. 99 per cent of the total under five mortality and maternal deaths are in the poor countries like South Asia and Sub-Saharan Africa. According to experts, if it progresses at the current pace, Sub-Saharan Africa will take not less than 150 years after 2015 to reduce child mortality by two-thirds. Figure 1 below is a projection regarding achieving the target set by MDG on the basis of recent performance of actual mortality rate[4].

Figure 1: Global Trends in Under-five Mortality, 1960-2000, with Projections to 2015

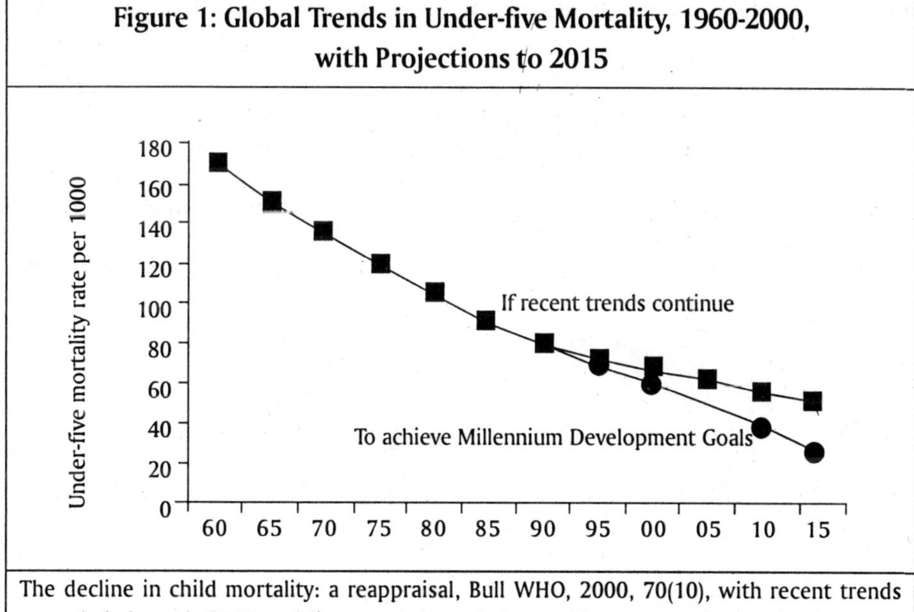

The decline in child mortality: a reappraisal, Bull WHO, 2000, 70(10), with recent trends extended through 2015 and linear trend needed to achieve a two-third reduction from 1990 levels.

Source: Make Every Mother and Child Count (WHO).

Some Measures of Child Health

One of the standard indicators of child health is Infant Mortality Rate (IMR)[5]. The world infant mortality rate has reduced to 83 in 2001 from 198 in 1960. OECD countries are also showing the same trend of low infant death. Though the infant mortality rates have declined considerably in less developed countries, the figures are still not satisfactory. The conditions of least developed nations are even worse. Sub-Saharan Africa has higher infant mortality and child mortality than South Asia. South Asia's performance is also a matter of concern.

The status of child health in an economy can also be measured in terms of immunization rate. The higher the immunization rate, it can be assumed that in that region, children are, in general, healthy. One of the indicators of achieving MDG 4 is Measles immunization coverage. According to a WHO Report it has increased from 47 per cent in 1958 to 77 per cent in 2005[6]. The global measles immunization shows an increasing trend (exceeds 75 per cent), but some regions (particularly, Sub-Saharan Africa and South Asia) are lagging behind. Figure 2 shows us a global picture region-wise.

Figure 2: Immunization Coverage with Measles Containing Vaccines for Infants, 2005

Measles immunization is one of the key indications to track progress towards the fourth Millennium Development Goal which aims to reduce, the mortality rate among children under five by two thirds. High coverage levels of routine immunization are needed to interrupt transmission and reduce child mortality.

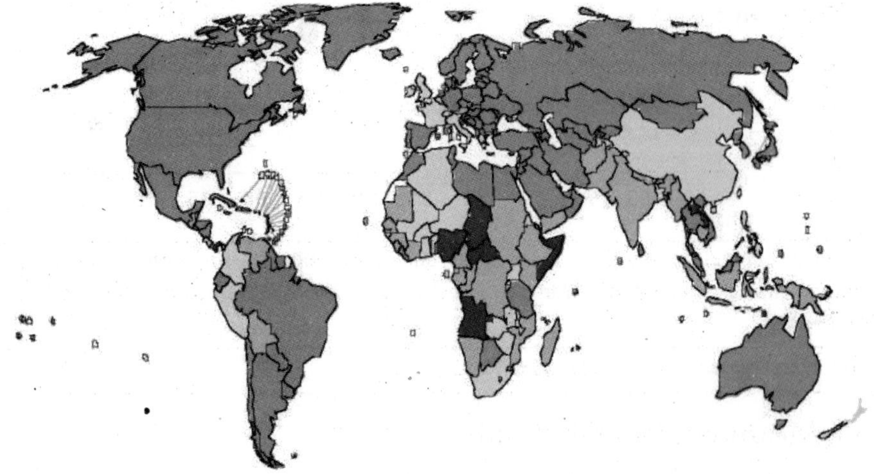

■ <50% (7 countries or territories, 4%)
■ 50-79% (31 countries or territories, 21%)
□ 80-89% (39 countries or territories, 20%)
■ >90% (106 countries or territories, 55%)

The boundaries and names shown and the designations used on this map do not imply the expression of any opinion whatsoever, on the part of the World Health Organization, concerning the legal status of any country, Territory, city or area or of its authorities, or concerning the delimitation of its frontiers or boundaries. Dotted lines on maps represent approximate border lines for which there may not yet be full agreement.

Source: WHO/UNICEF Coverage estimates 1980-2005, August 2006.

The number of infants being breastfed is another indicator of the society's effort to improve child health care services. Breastfeeding practice is being highly promoted in USA also. The National Health People 2010 of USA aimed to achieve the target of about 75 per cent of mothers initiating breastfeeding. In 2005, in 21 states of USA, 50 per cent mothers adopted breastfeeding practices for their child upto 6 months of age and in 11 states, 25 per cent mothers followed this practice upto 12 months of age[7].

However, the more worrying factor is that neonatal deaths (dying within the first four weeks) have increased in the developing countries. Some of the causes are the increasing age of mothers, the fertility treatments, etc. Again, undernutrition is considered to be one of the major causes responsible for more than half of deaths of children. Though Bangladesh has made a progress in terms of decline of underweight children from about 67 per cent to about 51 per cent from the period 1990-2000, the condition with respect to child malnutrition is severe. Underweight children are about half of the child population. Also, about 13 per cent to 19 per cent suffer from the problem of being severely stunted or underweight[8].

Factors Affecting Child Health

Experts are engaged in identifying the factors which are hindrances to the proper growth of a child. Apart from the income, which ensures the availability of adequate food, health care and nutrition are a few essential elements which a child requires for his balanced growth. The environment, in which a child is growing up, is also one of the most influential elements. Other elements, which according to experts, have a contributory role towards the total development of a child are – proper sanitation measures, clean surroundings, hygienic living conditions, etc. Parental education surely has a relation to the financial establishment of a family. A family, consisting of educated parents, is more likely to have a modest income, which, in turn, ensures the availability of adequate nutritious food. Also, the educated parents are expected to have more knowledge about healthy food habits, balanced diet, hygiene, proper sanitation measures, immunization measures available and the preventive measures to be taken for their child. Possibility of gender discrimination, being practiced mostly among illiterate segment of society, is expected to be low in educated families and hence it leads to healthier outcome in terms of proper birth spacing and number of children. Educated parents are expected to develop healthy food habits in their children. Hence the problem of overweight and obesity may be prevented.

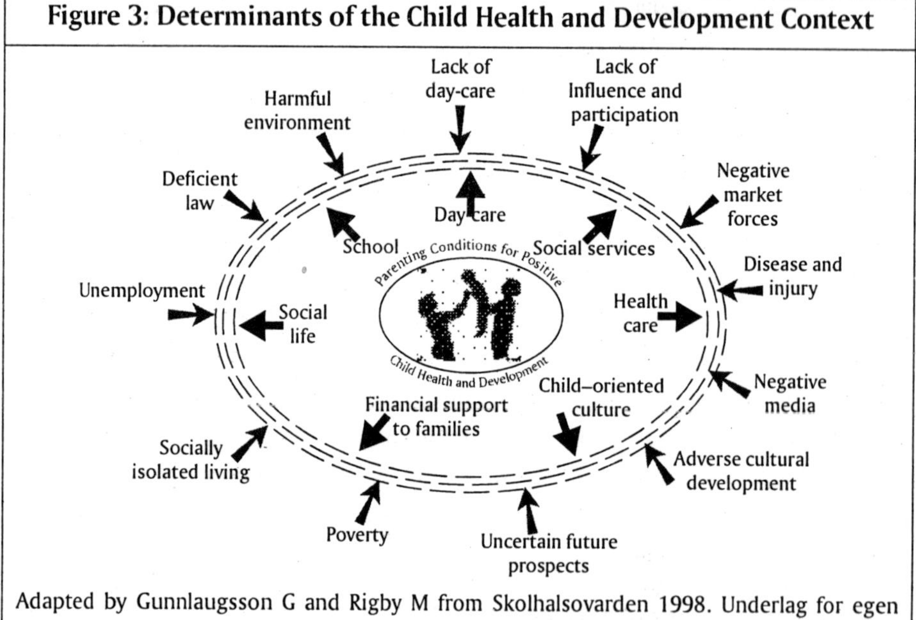

Figure 3: Determinants of the Child Health and Development Context

Adapted by Gunnlaugsson G and Rigby M from Skolhalsovarden 1998. Underlag for egen kontroll ochtillsyn. Stockholm: Socialstyrelsen. 1998.

Source: European Union Community Health Monitoring Programme: Child Health Indicators of Life and Development.

This figure is an attempt to identify factors which are affecting child health from the development perspectives.

Child Malnutrition

Malnutrition among children is one of the worst outcomes of child's ill health. It is a consequence of inadequate food, lack of care and occurs mostly due to diseases like diarrhea and pneumonia. It is the major cause of death of children worldwide. Deficiencies of iron, zinc, vitamins (A and B) are highly prevalent amongst children worldwide. South Asia ranks first, even higher than Sub-Saharan Africa, for malnutrition among children. India is the largest among them. Table 1 portrays the dismal situation in South Asia.

Poverty and Child Health

Studies have confirmed that health condition of a child depends on her socio-economic status. This is relevant for rich and poor countries as well as rich and poor households. Though the data on high income countries shows that 6 out of 1000

Table 1: Comparison between Countries of South Asia – Select Parameters of Development

Parameter	Bangladesh	India	Pakistan	Sri Lanka
Malnutrition in <5 years children (%)	56	53	26	34
Low birth weight (%)	30	33	25	34
Infant mortality rate	58	70	84	17
<5 mortality rate	89	98	112	19

Source: Early Nutrition and Health: Indian Perspective by Mahtab S Bamji.

children die before reaching 5 years of age. The poorest countries show the rate to be 120 out of 1000. In the developing countries, it is about 88 out of 1000 children. The gap between the rich and poor countries is increasing since there has been a reduction in under-five mortality of 71 per cent in the richer countries whereas it has been reduced by only 40 per cent in the poorer countries[9].

Worldwide, child mortality rate is showing different trends among high and low income households. In African countries a rising trend of child mortality is being observed in the poor families, whereas, a considerable improvement is prominent in case of economically well-off families. Such differences can be substantiated by factors like proper housing conditions, lack of adequate water and sanitation facilities, undernourished children due to lack of nutritional foods, etc. Low birth weight is also another disorder which resulted due to inadequate nutrition to mothers during their pregnancy or less age gap between the offspring. Coupled with these factors, there is also lack of immunization among poor children. These make poor children more prone to diseases. Even after getting sick, these poor children are not going to get proper health care facilities which only adds fuel to the problem. In addition to that, poor children are often found to be engaged in bad habits like smoking and other kinds of addiction due to the unhealthy living conditions. They are less likely to receive vaccinations and hence suffer from many preventable diseases.

Figure 4 shows the under 5 mortality rates of few developing countries (namely, Indonesia, Brazil, India, Kenya). The data has been segregated on the basis of the income of the households in these four countries. The figure validates the general trend of high mortality among poor countries. But the unusual fact is that in the case of Kenya and India the mortality rate is quite high even in the case of richer

Figure 4: Under-5 Mortality Rates by Socioeconomic Quintile of the Household for Selected Countries

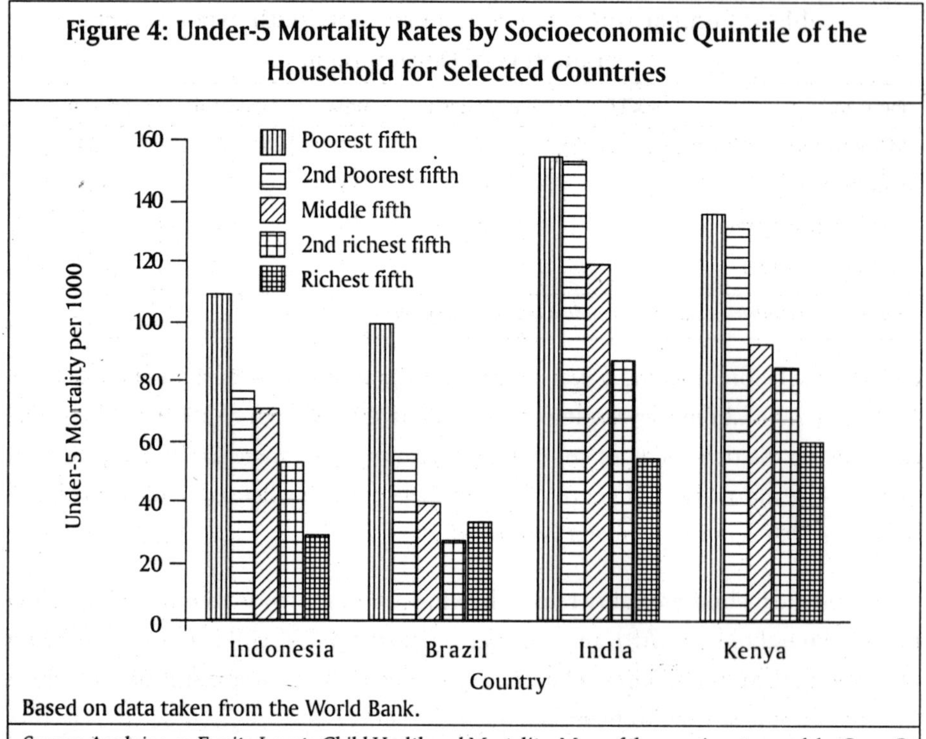

Based on data taken from the World Bank.

Source: Applying an Equity Lens to Child Health and Mortality: More of the same is not enough by Cesar G Victora, Adam Wagstaff, Joanna Armstrong Schellenberg, Davidson Gwatkin, Mariam Claeson, Jean-Pierre Habicht

households. Another message which we get from the figure is that the difference in mortality rate between the rich and the poor is considerably high in Indonesia and Brazil in comparison to India and Kenya.

Industrialization and Child Health

Rapid industrialization in the developing world shows that urban children are healthier than the children residing in the rural areas. The causes of this rural-urban disparity can be explained by factors like illiteracy, little or no knowledge about health care services and poor living standards in the rural areas. Factors like education of parents, child birth spacing, availability of proper sanitation and health facilities, safe drinking water, housing quality, cooking on stove rather than using wood or charcoal, provision of health care facilities etc., are major determinants. Urban regions characterized by industrialization signifies improved standard of living thus reducing the infant mortality rate. The rural-urban disparity is explained in terms of stunting which is a measure of the nutritional status and under-five mortality. Statistics reveal that about 33 per cent are stunted children in the developing countries. A survey conducted to measure the difference between rural and urban regions found that stunting and mortality is more prevalent among the poor. However, in countries like Bangladesh and Namibia, stunting is more in urban areas. Also mortality is more in Namibia and Paraguay. The reason can be urbanization which causes pollution and ill health[10].

Race, Gender and Child Health

Besides economic conditions, race and gender have a major stake in the case of child health. A survey conducted between black and white families in United States has shown that, there exists a higher rate of infant mortality among the black families. Asian children also are found to have poorer health conditions than the whites. However it is found that education of parents plays a major role in the health of their child. Asian and black families with lower educational backgrounds are found to have less healthy children than the white children. Effects of literacy on child health can also be judged from the fact that gender differences have an effect on child health. It is found generally that in places where gender differences in literacy rate are prominent, mortality rate is also high. Educated women have a better understanding about the health programmes (like public messages on vaccination, promotion of breastfeeding practices, immunization and other nutritional practices), the proper sanitation measures to be taken, sense of hygiene etc. Hence, they are more capable of taking care of their children rather than the illiterate mothers. An educated girl will probably marry at a higher age and will have proper family planning which result into necessary child spacing and enough knowledge about care and nutrition of the child. The literate women will be able to arrange food resources in the household in a way that the children have a balanced diet. Countries with gender differences like those of South Asia have lower literacy rates for women which in turn is a major factor for the ill health of children in these countries. A study on India reflects that gender differences exist even in terms of providing health care facilities. When sick, a boy child is more likely to be taken to the doctor rather than when a girl child falls sick. Also, immunization rates are higher for boys than girls. Malnourishment is more prevalent among girls rather than boys. Infant boys also are in an advantageous position with respect to breast feeding by their mothers compared to the girl child.

Figure 5: Child Mortality Rates in Males and Females in India

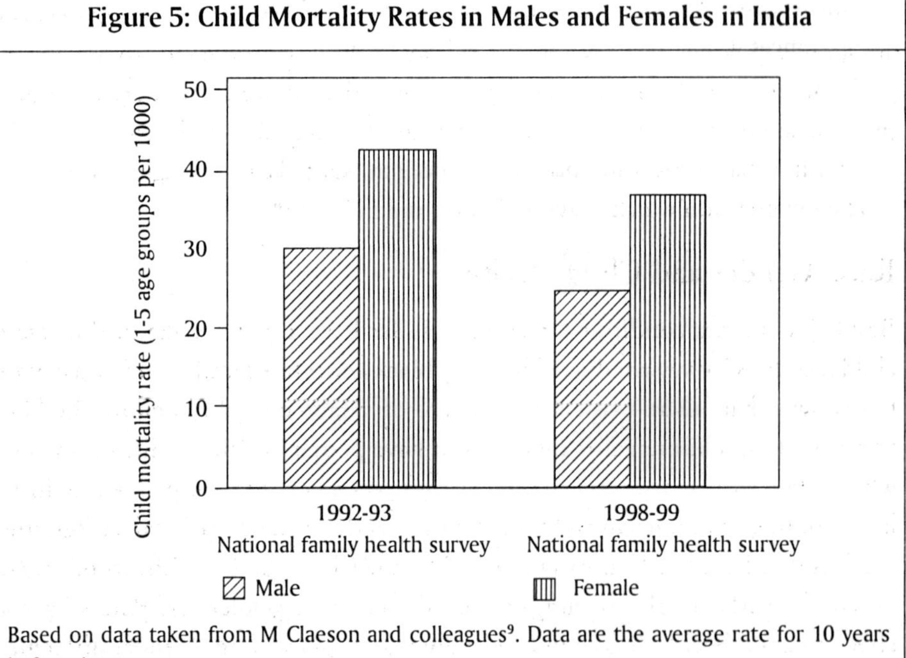

Based on data taken from M Claeson and colleagues[9]. Data are the average rate for 10 years before the survey.

Source: Applying an Equity Lens to Child Health and Mortality: More of the same is not enough by Cesar G Victora, Adam Wagstaff, Joanna Armstrong Schellenberg, Davidson Gwatkin, Mariam Claeson, Jean-Pierre Habicht

Child Labor and Health

Child Labor is against the freedom of the child. Though in situations of extreme poverty, child labour does add to the family's income and living standards, sometimes child's health concerns are being compromised by exposing them to hazardous situations. Toxic and harmful chemicals, pesticides and heavy machinery with huge noise pollution pose health risks to the child. Injuries like cuts and wounds, skin problems, psychological problems are some of the risks, faced by a child who joins the labour force. Studies have revealed that children absorb more of the chemicals in their blood and tissues given that, both adults and children are exposed to the same amount of chemicals. Long working hours for children cause malnutrition and fatigue due to inadequate food intake and stress. Children become victims of hearing loss due to the noise levels at their workplace which are above the permissible range. Since children are more sensitive to heat, the heat standards maintained in many of the work places may be very harmful to their health. Usually children are made to work in fatal and unhealthy circumstances where adults normally would avoid working and that too at low wage.

Steps Taken Globally

History tells us that in the past, policy makers adopted mainly disease-specific, technology-dependent policy reform, which was expected to deliver dramatic figures within a very short span of time. Malaria Eradication Programme (initiated in 1950s and discarded in 1970s) is an example of such initiatives. Though it was not exclusively focused on children, it was expected to contribute significantly in decreasing the infant mortality rate.

In 1977, World Health Assembly "health for all by the year 2000" goal had been adopted by the member countries. This was characterized as more people-centric and community-based, where the focal point was the primary health care services. Programmatic areas had been emphasized instead of specific disease under this policy reform. Under this programme emphasis has been given to the equitable distribution of resources to few identified factors (like improved water supplies, proper sanitation,

Figure 6: Proportion of Government Subsidies to the Health Sector that Effectively Reaches the Poorest and Richest 20% of Families

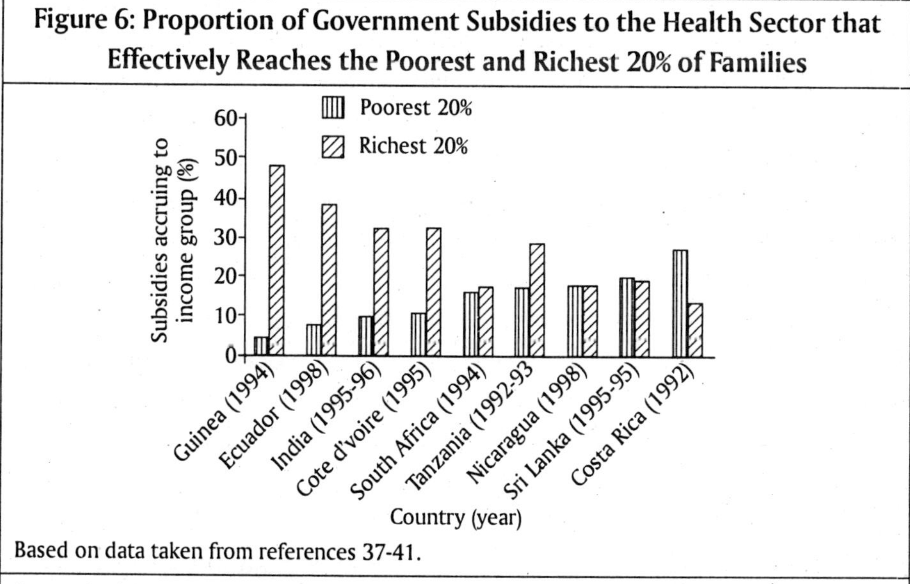

Based on data taken from references 37-41.

Source: Applying an Equity Lens to Child Health and Mortality: More of the same is not enough by Cesar G Victora, Adam Wagstaff, Joanna Armstrong Schellenberg, Davidson Gwatkin, Mariam Claeson, Jean-Pierre Habicht

healthy environment, family planning etc.) which have a positive influence towards the overall development of a child.

This strategy focuses on the disease identified, which is the major contributor to the increased mortality rate. This approach seems to be more focused and feasible. Under this strategy, policy-maker would be able to channel the resources to the focused areas which is expected to deliver demonstrable success in a short span of time. According to data, children are most vulnerable to preventable diseases. This is one of the key reasons why policy planners thought that this strategy would be the most effective one.

Figure 6 gives a real picture of the actual proportion of government subsidies reaching the poorest sector of the society in a few developing countries.

Few Interventions by Some International Organizations

The World Health Organization (WHO) first initiated expanded programme on immunization and then the Programme for the Control of Diarrhoeal Diseases. Parallely, UNICEF initiated intervention on issues like – growth monitoring, oral rehydration therapy, breastfeeding promotion, and immunization, popularly known as GOBI. Later on, three more issues have been added – female education, family planning and food. Different governments started channelising funds in different regions-specific child survival programmes which have a root in community based approach. Another similar approach is the Integrated Management of Childhood Illness. This programme has a component of community development. It has been evolved from some selective primary health care programmes which have been aimed to put a check on diarrhoeal diseases and acute respiratory infections. Countries like Afghanistan, Nigeria, India and Pakistan, Somalia, Kenya, Ethiopia, Indonesia, Namibia, Angola, Bangladesh, Cameroon, Democratic Republic of Congo, Yemen need concentrated efforts to eradicate polio. CDC (Centers for Disease Control and Prevention) along with WHO and UNICEF and Rotary International have joined hands to work for the eradication of polio.

Conclusion

While formulating a health programme, policy-makers generally not only take care of issues like financial resources but they also consider behavioral aspects and role of community in the whole programme. Ultimately, the core emphasis should be on the development of a an organized healthcare delivery system, so that the required health care services reach to the level of the society which need these facilities most.

But in spite of the above facts – none of the above strategies work completely. Though the malaria eradication programme was unable to bring the expected results, smallpox eradication programme was a grand success. With this fact it has been proved that the success of such health programmes lies in the participation and adoptability of the community. It would be ideal, if the lessons learnt from the successful and failed programmes can be incorporated in the future programmes.

(Dalia Dey is an M.Sc. in Economics from University of Calcutta and MBA in Financial Management from Indian Institute of Social Welfare and Business Management, Kolkata and member of the editorial team, Icfai Research Centre, Kolkata and

Kasturi Nandy is an MA in Economics from Jadavpur University and member of the editorial team of Icfai Research Centre, Kolkata.)

Endnotes

1 *http://en.wikipedia.org/wiki/Infant_mortality*

2 *http://www.unausa.org*

3 *http://www.cdc.gov*

4 Make Every Mother and Child Count: World Health Organization.

5 Infant Mortality Rate-Probability of dying between birth and exactly one year of age expressed per 1,000 live births. (Source: *www.unicef.org*).

6 Immunization Summary: The 2007 Edition by UNICEF & WHO.

7 *http://www.cdc.gov/breastfeeding/data/NIS_data/data_2005.htm*

8 Millennium Development Goals: Bangladesh Progress Report, 2005.

9 Applying an equity lens to child health and mortality: more of the same is not enough by Cesar G Victora, Adam Wagstaff, Joanna Armstrong Schellenberg, Davidson Gwatkin, Mariam Claeson, Jean-Pierre Habicht.

10 Are urban children really healthier? Evidence from 47 developing countries by Ellen Van de Poela, Owen O'Donnellab and Eddy Van Doorslaerac.

References

Early nutrition and health: Indian Perspective, Author: Mahtab S Bamji, October 2003 *www.ias.ac.in/currsci/oct252003/1137*

"Make Every Mother and Child Count: World Health Organization" *http://www.who.int/world-health-day*

Countdown to 2015: Tracking Progress in Child Survival (*http://welcometotheMillennium CampaignNewsCenter-MillenniumCampaign.htm*).

"Child and Adolescent Health and Development: e-Update December",. 2006 *http://www.who.int/topics/child_health/en*

The evolution of child health programmes in developing countries: from targeting diseases to targeting people. Author: Mariam Claeson1 & Ronald J Waldman (*http://whqlibdoc.who.int/bulletin/2000/Number%2010/78(10)1234-1245.pdf*).

Poverty Experience, Race, and Child Health, Authors: Jennifer Malat, Hyun Joo Oh, Mary Ann Hamilton (*www.publichealthreports.org/userfiles/120_4/120442.pdf*).

Understanding health disparities: The Role of race and socio-economic status in children's health, Authors: Edith Chen, Andrew D Martin, Karen A Matthews (*www.ajph.org/cgi/content/full/96/4/702*).

Toxic Chemicals and Childhood Cancer: A Review of the Evidence, 2003, Authors: Tami Gouveia-Vigeant and Joel Tickner.

Child labour and Health: Evidence and Research Issues, 2002. Author: O O Donnell, E Van Doorslaer, F Rosati.

Applying an equity lens to child health and mortality: more of the same is not enough, Authors: Cesar G Victora, Adam Wagstaff, Joanna Armstrong Schellenberg, Davidson Gwatkin, Mariam Claeson, Jean-Pierre Habicht.

Child Health Indicators of Health and Development, Authors: Michael Rigby and Lennart Kohler.

"Child Poverty in perspective: An Overview of child well being in rich countries". UNICEF, 2007.

Health and Millennium Development Goals, WHO 2005.

"Child Labor and Health: Adult Education Workshop", The University of IOWA.

"Are urban children really healthier? Evidence from 47 developing countries by Ellen Van de Poela", Owen O'Donnellab and Eddy Van Doorslaerac.

Millenium Development Goals: Bangladesh Progress Report, 2005.

4

Behaviour Development in Babies
Its Improvement in Relation with Ecological Factors

Bimla Dhanda and Sudha Chhikara

The infants' early interaction experiences are determined by a multitude of biological, cultural and environmental factors. If the performance of infants in a particular development is declining that may be improved by improving his home environment or enforcement by intervention programme. In view of the above, present investigation was undertaken to identify the developmental deficiencies in babies with reference to social skill development, to delineate the crucial ecological factors affecting this development, and to study the impact of intervention programme on social skills development. Present study was conducted at two locations, viz., Hisar city as urban and Rawalwas Klan and Siswal villages as rural. The purposes of selection of localities were easy accessibility and rapport with the respondents. Totally 400 babies in the age group of 12-24 months were selected randomly for investigation. The sample was divided into four age groups, viz., 12-15, 15-18, 18-21 and 21-24 months, and over the localities and gender. Thus, there were 25 male and 25 female babies in each age group.

Source: www.krepublishers.com, Journal of Human Ecology Vol. 19, Issue 3 pp. 215-219, March 2006.

Significant differences for all the age groups were observed for all the variables. This indicated that formation of different age groups at the interval of 3 months for these variables was appropriate. In social skill development, males, in general, were better than females. Interaction of age x gender also revealed that the boys learned social skills differently than girls over the different age groups. Comparison of urban and rural sample also revealed that urban babies, in general were better than rural in social skills development. Regarding associations with economic factors, it appeared that the babies from higher income group generally had better development in social skills under both urban and rural areas. Intervention proved highly effective for development of social skills in both urban and rural areas.

Introduction

A human infant's attachment becomes apparent through discrete observable behaviour such as smiling and crying, which are deemed to possess a signalling function that serves to activate maternal behaviour and bring the adult into proximity to the child. Rooting, grasping, sucking, following, approaching, clinging are behaviours whereby the infant plays an active role in seeking proximity and contact. As from birth these behaviours become coordinated and focused on the mother to form the basis of attachment. In any case, the infant becomes attached to the caregiver with whom he has had more interaction, generally his mother (Cooper et al. 2002). When the child achieves locomotion a new behaviour becomes activated, that of exploratory behaviour. Exploration of the environment is antithetical to attachment. It is of the utmost importance to focus the relationship of the infant to his mother as keeping a balance in the interplay between both systems.

One of the most important functions of the attachment behavioural system is to intervene in the baby's excursions into the environment, in response to a variety of potentially dangerous events, thereby deactivating the exploratory system and activating the attachment system thus seeking proximity to his mother. Several studies show that children approach their caregivers not only in response to dangerous external stimuli but also they do so to check the availability and attentiveness of the caregiver, in a sort of permanent monitoring activity. After such checking the child wanders off to play again; after a while he returns again, and so on. This kind of behavioural pattern is referred to in the literature as the baby using his mother as a Secure Base (Ainsworth et al., 1978).

Infants tried facial expressions, vocalizations and body movements to get their mothers to respond again. When these efforts failed they reacted to their mothers' sad, vacant gaze by turning away, frowning and crying (Ellsworth et al., 1993; Gusella et al., 1988; Mayes and Carter, 1990). By the end of the first year, infants deliberately look to others for emotional cues and evaluate uncertain events, such as, the approach of a stranger. Since, infants cannot describe their feelings, researchers face challenging tasks determining exactly which emotions they are experiencing. Although vocalizations and body movements provide some information, facial expressions seem to offer the most reliable cue during the age of 18-24 months (Mc Donald, 1997).

Cross-cultural evidence indicates that when infants are looking at photographs of different facial gestures, people around the world associate them with emotions in the same way. In the 1970s and 1980s, the pragmatic movements in the field of speech-language pathology influenced by social-cognitive learning theory re-established the idea that language is embedded in a social matrix. This movement taught us that children do not talk about objects of interest in isolation. They communicate in the context of social interactions often for socially and emotionally driven reasons (Klein and Mosses, 1994). This orientation underscored the importance of care-giver-child interactions for language development and broadened our awareness of the range of issues that need to be considered in language intervention. Social and environmental factors have become so intricately related to health and diseases that often care must go beyond medical intervention. Child developmentalists have partially succeeded in designing and implementing early childhood intervention programmes to ameliorate social aspects of childhood morbidity.

Interventions and impact studies offer a wide variation in goals, coverage, theoretical assumptions and research designs. Most studies, carried out in the seventies and eighties, are empirical in nature. A substantive analysis of these studies indicates that a wide range of dimensions, mainly language, cognitive and social development have been studied, thus, opening a large area for future research and action. Another crucial point is that many intervention evaluation studies lack a theoretical base in terms of the relationship between the organism and the environment (Gottfried, 1983). Such an approach may prove useful in gaining deeper insight into alternative intervention strategies appropriate for different groups of children.

The intervention may act directly on children by including new capacities and programmes in individuals or may attempt to modify the behaviour of various people, institutions or media that influences the lives of children (Gholson and Rosenthal, 1984). In view of this, the present study was undertaken with the objectives, namely, to identify the developmental deficiencies in babies for social development, to delineate the crucial ecological factors and to study the impact of intervention programmes affecting social development of babies.

Materials and Methods

Present study was conducted at two locations, viz., Hisar city as urban and Rawalwas Klan and Siswal villages as rural. The purposes of selection of localities were easy accessibility and rapport with the respondents. Totally, 400 babies during the age of 12-24 months were selected randomly for investigation. The sample was divided into four age groups, viz., 12-15, 15-18, 18-21 and 21-24 months, and over the localities and gender. Thus, there were 25 male and 25 female babies in each age group. These data were collected in two phases. During phase I the babies were observed for social skills by Vineland Scales of Social Maturity (Sparrow et al., 1984). In addition, data on family income were also observed.

During phase II the deficient group of babies for social development was identified on the basis of the mean performance of the babies. Thus, the intervention programme on home based techniques was developed for each age group for all the domains under study. Before administering the intervention, the programme was assessed by the team of learned scientists of College of Home Science, CCS HAU, Hisar as well as from other institutions. All the necessary suggestions were incorporated. The intervention programme was first applied on a part of sample and its effects were assessed. Then all the items were scrutinised carefully and some unimportant items were dropped. Intervention was finally applied for a period of one month.

Results and Discussion

Social development of babies starts in early life and by the end of second year, self recognition is well established and underlines children's first struggle with peers over objects, personal acts and formation of a categorical self (Berk, 1996). Analysis of variance revealed that social skills of babies differed significantly over the age groups in urban (F = 5.71*) and in rural (F = 17.83**) areas (Table 1). Mean squares for gender in urban (F = 14.44**) and in rural (F = 6.05**) areas were also significant. The interaction between age x gender was significant only in urban area (F = 4.50**). When the mean values of males and females were compared, it was found that means of females (97.85±2.86) were higher than males (89.14±3.67) in urban (F=14.44**) area (Table 2). Similar trend was found in rural area. Significant Z values for all the age groups as well as for overall means, revealed that mean values of rural babies were higher than urban babies in all the age groups (Z = 6.95**).

Table 1: Analysis of Variance for Social Skills of Babies during the Age of One to Two Years

Source of variation	D.f.	SS	MS	F
Urban				
Age	3	4489.18	1496.39	5.71**
Gender	1	3784.50	3784.50	14.44**
Age X Gender	3	3538.37	1179.46	4.50**
Error	192	50336.64	262.17	
Total	199	62148.69		
Rural				
Age	3	11403.06	3801.02	17.83**
Gender	1	1290.32	1290.32	6.05*
Age X Gender	3	1332.62	377.54	1.77
Error	192	40930.56	213.18	
Total	199	54756.56		

*, **: Significant at 5% and 1% level of significance, respectively.

Table 2: Means and Standard Deviations of Social Skills Domain for Children during the Age One to Two Years

Gender	Age in months				
	12-15	15-18	18-21	21-24	Pooled Mean
Urban					
Boys	80.55	86.45	90.15	99.50	89.14
	(4.20)	(2.92)	(3.60)	(3.52)	(3.67)
Girls	90.25	105.45	100.50	95.20	97.85
	(3.10)	(2.00)	(2.90)	(3.85)	(2.86)
Pooled Mean	85.40	95.95	95.33	97.35	93.51
	(3.52)	(2.61)	(3.21)	(3.62)	(3.11)
Rural					
Boys	90.50	98.50	105.15	110.20	101.09
	(4.75)	(4.65)	(3.10)	(2.96)	(3.15)
Girls	96.35	100.15	117.65	110.50	106.16
	(3.65)	(2.38)	(3.45)	(2.13)	(2.73)
Pooled Mean	93.43	99.33	111.40	110.35	103.63
	(3.57)	(3.17)	(3.25)	(2.24)	(2.81)
Z test for Urban vs Rural	11.28**	5.82**	24.88**	21.59**	6.95**

Figures in parentheses denote standard deviations,

**: Significant at 1% level of significance.

In the present study babies showed significant differences in development of social development skills for all the age groups. Females were better than males in social skills. This revealed the natural instinct the babies had in their respective fields. Morriset et al. (1995) also found that girls were better than boys in social development during the age of 20 to 30 months. Similarly, Crandell, and Hobson (1999) found significant differences in various aspects of social development in different socio-economic groups. They also found that social development of babies was related to parent-child relationship and intellectual development of babies. The interaction of gender with different intervals of age group revealed that differences were observed for development of social skills only in urban areas. Social development was an important predictor of personality development and closely related with social-life abilities (Sun et al., 1997). In addition, study of social development of babies is important particularly during first year of life because it is the period of emerging self and shaping children for predominant modes of viewing and experiencing world (Mayes and Cohen, 1993). Among different domains of social development, social skills had significant impact because these skills contribute to behaviour for human social interactions. During the age of 12 months, the infants become sensitive to self and perceptual features of other objects mainly inanimate objects (Pipp-Siegel and Foltz, 1997).

As a whole, there was a significant increase in all the activities of social development after every three months of interval. As usual the social development of urban babies was better than of rural babies. Interaction effects revealed that boys and girls learn social development differently.

Impact of Intervention Programme

Constructing an intervention programme is as much an art as a science, requiring a creative interplay between existing cultural and political realities, prevailing scientific theories and paradigms and the research data applicable to the processes or deficits to be modified. The task of this investigation was to explore methods for preventing developmental deficiencies. In order to complete this task the current knowledge of theory and research pertaining to home environment and various developments of babies were examined. Finally, workable intervention strategies were devised and evaluated by learned experts.

Intervention programme had significant impact on social skills development. Mays and Cohen (1993) said that it is an important period for improvement of social abilities of babies. Because during this period, personality of child may be shaped, refined and remodeled in the context of loving relations. Sun et al. (1997) also reported that early period of childhood is an important period for personality of children to be developed towards extroversion tendencies. Therefore, social learning aspect should be an important component of child's learning process (Lutjein et al., 1998). In order to develop an intervention programme for developing social skills in babies the positive emotion of children should be taken care of and false belief on the parts of parents (Watson et al., 1999). In addition, parental involvement and avoidance of negative emotions should also be an important tool

Table 3: Effect of Intervention Programme on Social Skills of Babies during the Age of One to Two Years

Variable/	No. of babies	Mean of babies before intervention	Mean of babies after intervention	Mean of babies in control	% of increase over control	t test control vs inter-vention
Urban						
12-15	130(3.25)	60.78±1.25	96.35±1.17	62.75±0.85	53.55	51.95**
15-18	110(2.75)	65.35±2.78	94.40±2.86	63.70±4.65	48.19	12.57**
18-21	110(2.75)	60.15±3.95	99.30±3.05	69.85±3.90	42.16	13.30**
21-24	100(2.50)	67.79±2.86	97.15±1.96	73.20±4.37	32.72	11.18**
Total/Pooled mean	45(11.25)	63.52±3.67	96.80±2.03	47.38±5.00	43.66	20.48**
Rural						
12-15	120(3.00)	56.17±2.68	86.10±3.96	59.15±1.18	45.50	14.58**
15-18	130(3.25)	54.87±3.70	90.15±1.75	61.10±1.91	47.55	25.08**
18-21	160(4.00)	59.69±2.61	85.70±3.65	60.75±1.10	41.07	14.63**
21-24	140(3.50)	60.17±1.93	92.65±1.10	62.35±0.75	45.71	50.89**
Total/Pooled mean	55(13.75)	57.73±2.61	88.65±3.34	60.84±1.32	45.71	17.32**

Figures in parentheses denote percentages; ?± values indicate standard deviations.
*, **: Significant at 5% and 1% level of significance, respectively.

Table 4: Association of Economic Status of the Family with Social Skills of Babies during the Age of One to Two Years

	Urban					Rural				
	H	M	L	Total	χ^2	H	M	L	Total	χ^2
H	21 (38.2)	22 (40.0)	12 (21.8)	55		27 (42.9)	26 (41.3)	10 (15.8)	63	
M	26 (32.5)	38 (47.5)	16 (20.0)	80		18 (24.7)	41 (56.2)	14 (19.2)	73	
L	20 (30.8)	24 (36.9)	21 (32.3)	65		11 (17.2)	23 (35.9)	30 (46.9)	64	
Total	67	84	49	200	1.81	56	90	54	200	27.73**

*, **: Significant at 5% and 1%, respectively; Figures in parentheses represent percentages.
H, M, L: Denote high, medium and low categories, respectively.

for improvement of social development of babies (Iurko et al., 1999). Parental reactions to children's negative emotions and socially appropriate behaviour of children were the important aspects in the improvement of social behaviour of babies (Eisenberg et al., 1999).

Impact of Economic Status on Social Skills Development

The aim of the intervention was to provide the mother with emotional support and to encourage her in sensitive responsive interactions with her infant. A major aspect of the intervention was the use of particular items from the manuals prepared for the purpose. Family income appeared to be the important variable as it was associated with development of social skills. This may be attributed to better nutrition, play material, care and involvement with children in high income group Bradly and Caldwell (1984). Similarly in a study of 12 to 24 months old babies, Gottfried (1983) observed that SES was positively related with various parameters of child development and particularly with cognitive development. Wachs (1984) also reported that family income was closely related with developmental parameters of babies.

As a whole, there was a significant increase in all the activities of social development after every three months of interval. As usual the social development of urban babies was better than of rural babies. Interaction effects revealed that boys and girls learn social development differently. Therefore, more emphasis should be given in rural area to improve the status of rural babies.

(Bimla Dhanda and Sudha Chhikara, Department of Human Development and Family Studies, College of Home Science, CCS Haryana Agricultural University, Hisar, Haryana, India.)

References

Ainsworth, M.D.S., Blehar, M.C., Waters, E. and Wall, S.: Platters of attachment: A psychological study of the strong situation. Erlbaum, Hilside, N.J. (1978).

Berk, L. E.: *Child Development.* Prentice, Hall of India, New Delhi (1996).

Bradley, R. H. and Caldwell, B. M.: A study of the relationship between home environment and cognitive development during first five years. In: A. W. Gottfried. (Ed.): *Home Environment and Early Cognitive Development.* Academic Press, N. Y. (1984).

Cooper, P. J., Landman, N., Tomlinson, M., Molteno, Mark and Swartz, L.: Impact of a mother—infant intervention in an indigent peri-urban South African context. *The British Journal of Psychiatry,* 180: 76-81 (2002).

Crandell, L. E. and Hobson, R. P.: Individual diferences in young children's I. Q: A social-developmental perspective. *J. Child Psychol. Psychiatry,* 40(3): 455-464 (1999).

Eisenberg, N., Fabes, R. A., Shepard, S. A., Guthrie, I. K., Murphy, B.C. and Reiser, M.: Parental relations to children's negative emotions: Longitudinal relations to quality of children's social functioning. *Child Dev.,* 70(2): 513-534 (1999).

Ellsworth, C. P., Muir, D. W. and Hains, S. M.: Social competence and person - object differentiations: An analysis of still face effect. *Dev. Psychol.,* 29: 73-87 (1993).

Gottfried, A. W.: Measures of socio-economic measures in child development research: Data and presentations. *Presented at Biennial Convention for the Society for Research in Child Development,* Detroit (1983).

Gholson, B. and Rosenthal, T. L.: *Applications of Cognitive Development Theory.* Academic Press, New York (1984).

Gusella, J. L., Muir, D. W. and Tornick, E. Z.: The effect of manipulating maternal behaviour during an interaction on 3 and 6 - month - olds effect and attention. *Child Dev.,* 59: 1111-1124 (1988).

Iurko, G. P., Terent, G. V., Ivanova, O. G., Veremkovich, L. V., Lashneva, I. P., Berezina, N. O. and Latkina, L. I.: Increasing of functional abilities of preschool children by means of physical Training. *Vestn Ross. Akad. Med. Nauk.,* 6: 7-13 (1999).

Klein, H. B. and Moses, N.: *Intervention Planning for Children With Communication Disorders: A Guide for Clinical Practicum and Professional Practice.* Prentice Hall, New Jersey (1994).

Luteijn, E., Jackson, S., Volkmar, F. R. and Minderaa, R. B.: The development of the children's social behaviour questionnaire. *J. Antism Dev. Disord.,* 28(6): 559-565 (1998).

Mays, L. C. and Carter, A. S.: Emerging social regulatory capacities as seen in the still face situation. *Child Dev.,* 61: 754-763 (1990).

Mays, L. C. and Cohen, D. J.: The social matrix of aggression: Enactment and representation of learning and hating in the first year of life. *Psychonal. Study Child.,* 48: 145-169 (1993).

Mc Donald, J. L.: Language acquisition: The acquisition of linguistic structure in normal and special populations. *Ann. Rev. Psychol.,* 48: 215-241 (1997).

Morriset, C. E., Barnard, K. E. and Booth, C. I.: Toddlers language development: Sex differences within social risk. *Dev. Psychol.*, 31: 851-865 (1995).

Pipp-Siegel, S. and Foltz, C.: Toddlers acquisition of self/other knowledge. *Child Dev.*, 68(1): 69-79 (1997).

Sparrow, S. S., Balla, D. A. and Cicchetti, D. V.: *Vineland Adaptive Behaviour Scales.* AGS Circle Pines, Minnesota, USA (1984).

Sun, R., Zhang, Q. and Shang, C.: Study on relationship between personality traits and social life. *Chung Hua. Hu. Li. Tsa. Chih.*, 32(3): 135-137 (1997).

Wachs, T. D.: Proximal experience and early cognitive-intellectual development. In: A. W. Gottfried. (Ed.): *Home Environment and Early Cognitive Development.* Academic Press, N. Y. (1984).

Watson, A. W.: Height, body weight, skinfold thickness and endurance fitness of children attending national schools in Ireland. *Jr. J. Med. Sci.*, 162(9): 358-361 (1993).

5

Malnutrition and the Developing Mind

Bhoomika Rastogi Kar, Shobini L Rao and B A Chandramouli

Malnutrition is associated with both structural and functional pathology of the brain. A wide range of cognitive deficits has been reported in malnourished children. Effect of chronic protein energy malnutrition (PEM) causing stunting and wasting in children could also affect the ongoing development of higher cognitive processes during childhood (> 5 years of age). The present study examines the effect of stunted growth on the rate of development of cognitive processes using neuropsychological measures. Development of cognitive processes appeared to be governed by both age and nutritional status. Malnourished children performed poor on tests of attention, working memory, learning and memory and visuo spatial ability except on the test of motor speed and coordination. Chronic protein energy malnutrition (stunting) affects the ongoing development of higher cognitive processes during childhood years rather than merely showing a generalized cognitive impairment. Stunting could result in slowing in the age related improvement in certain and not all higher order cognitive processes and may also result in long lasting cognitive impairments.

Introduction

Depending on its intensity and duration, nutritional deficiency can disrupt the structure and function of the nervous system of humans. Malnutrition is associated with both structural and functional pathology of the brain. Structurally malnutrition results in tissue damage, growth retardation, disorderly differentiation, reduction in synapses and synaptic neurotransmitters, delayed myelination and reduced overall development of dendritic arborization of the developing brain. Malnutrition affects brain and cognitive development. Developing mind is sensitive to the effects of brain damage caused by malnutrition. There are deviations in the temporal sequences of brain maturation, which in turn disturb the formation of neuronal circuits [1].

Malnutrition is also associated with a wide range of cognitive deficits also reported by Indian studies. In India malnutrition is a serious concern. WHO report states that for the years 1990-1997 52% of Indian children less than 5 years of age suffered from severe to moderate malnutrition [2]. Malnourished children show poor development in all areas of behaviour i.e., motor, adaptive, language and personal social [3]. Rural children studying in primary school between the ages of 6-8 years were assessed on measures of social maturity, visuo-motor co-ordination, and memory. Malnutrition is associated with deficits of social competence, visuo-motor coordination and memory. Malnutrition affects immediate memory of boys more as compared to those of girls. Delayed recall of words and pictures of malnourished boys has been found to be impaired. Malnourished girls had an impairment of delayed recall of only words. IQ scores have been found to decrease with the severity of malnutrition. Performance IQ has been found to be affected more than the verbal IQ as well as on the subtests of information and digit span among the verbal subtests [4]. The above study has shown that though there could be a decrease in full scale IQ, yet performance on all the subtests may not be affected. Malnutrition may affect different neuropsychological functions to different degrees.

Development of the Brain and Mind

Brain development and cognitive maturation occur concurrently during childhood and adolescence. Developmental neuroimaging has provided data on postnatal structural and functional maturation of the brain-from childhood to adolescence. Structural maturation of brain regions and connections determines cognitive development to certain extent. However, less clear-cut relationships have been observed between development of brain structure and cognitive development. Brain continues to undergo major changes after birth— throughout childhood and adolescence [5-6]. Brain growth is marked by neurodevelopmental events such as neuronal density, dendritic growth, synaptic density and myelination. Cortical changes between childhood & adolescence are confined to dorsal regions prominently front al and parietal cortices, which is related to improved cognitive abilities [6]. Brain growth occurs in spurts showing a change at irregular intervals approximately every two years [7]. Myelination is a neurodevelopmental event, which continues until adolescence and has shown different rates of maturation across different brain regions. Ongoing process of myelination is related to the formation of networks and development of higher cognitive functions in childhood & adolescence [8].

The sequence in which the cortex matures parallels the cognitive milestones. Primary sensory, somatosensory and motor areas are advanced at birth followed by parietal and temporal association areas associated with language and spatial skills and higher order association areas such as prefrontal cortex associated with top down control of attention and other cognitive functions are the last to mature [9-10]. Prefrontal functions have shown differential performance and improvement over 4-7 years [11] and 8-10 years continuing up to 12 years of age [12].

Different functional systems develop at different rates. Some reports suggest that cognitive functions such as attention, fluency, working memory, and response inhibition develop rapidly between 5-8 years and at a more moderate rate between 9-12 years [13]. Some studies report a significant change between 8-10 years as compared to 11-13 years of age [14]. A recent study by Waber and colleagues carried out in the US reported a rapid and early maturation (6-10 years) of neuropsychological functions. They also observed a decline in performance from 10-12 years until 16 years of age. They found that children achieve adult levels of performance by 10-12 years of age. They conclude that the developmental trends are rapid in the early years and slowly level off by 12 years and further start declining until 16 years of age [15]. Developmental trajectories across the various cognitive domains are quite heterogeneous which also implies that there could be variable extents of effects of environmental stressors like malnutrition on the rapid ongoing postnatal brain and cognitive development.

Malnutrition and Brain Development

The early formative years of rapid brain and cognitive development are sensitive to adverse effects of many factors like malnutrition. Our conceptions of how malnutrition occurring early in life affects brain development have evolved since the mid-1960s. At that time, it was believed that malnutrition during certain critical periods in early development would result in brain damage possibly in mental retardation and impairment in brain function. We now know that most of the alterations in the growth of various brain structures eventually recover, although permanent alterations in certain regions like hippocampus and cerebellum remain. However, recent research has shown long-lasting, changes in brain function resulting from malnutrition [16].

Neuropsychological Dysfunction and Malnutrition

Neuropsychology is the study of brain behaviour relationships. A neuropsychological evaluation informs us about the functional status of the brain affected by malnutrition. Deficits of cognitive, emotional and behavioural functioning are linked to structural abnormalities of different regions of the brain. Brain structures and brain circuits compute different components of cognitive operations [17]. Neuropsychological assessment is a noninvasive method to measure brain functioning. The differential nature of cognitive deficits further suggests that different areas of the brain are affected to different degrees. A Neuropsychological assessment helps to delineate the pattern of brain dysfunction and to identify the topography of brain damage. Malnourishment is a grave problem in our country. The fact that it affects the developing brain and mind makes it even more a serious issue to attend to in terms of providing better health services as preventive measures and some kind to cognitive rehabilitation once the deficits have occurred.

We conducted a study as a preliminary step to investigate the nature of brain dysfunction and delay in the development of cognitive functions through neuropsychological assessment in malnourished children [18]. 20 adequately nourished children and 20 malnourished children in the age range of 5–10 years going to normal schools in the city of Bangalore participated in the study. Children studying in a corporation school were screened for malnourishment. Stunting and wasting were taken as indicators of moderate to severe malnutrition. In each parameter the 50th percentile was considered to be normal and less than 2 standard deviation from the median was indicative of moderate to severe malnutrition. Only those children who were stunted or those who were both stunted and wasted were included in the malnourished group.

Coloured progressive matrices test [19] was administered to rule out mental retardation. The Children's Behaviour Questionnaire Form B [20] was administered to the class teachers of the identified children. A large percentage of children from the malnourished group as well as the adequately nourished group (92% and 89% respectively) came from low socio economic status.

Both the groups were assessed on the NIMHANS neuropsychological battery for children [21] to examine neuropsychological functions such as motor speed, attention, speech, executive functions, visuospatial functions, learning, memory and comprehension. Malnourished group performed poor on tests of fluency, attention, working memory, visuospatial functions, verbal comprehension and learning and memory. Their performance was adequate on tests of motor speed and expressive speech.

Cognitive deficits associated with malnutrition have been reported in the past. However, neuropsychological dysfunction associated with malnutrition has not been studied so much. Performance has been found to be poor on all the neuropsychological functions except that on motor speed and expressive speech. Malnourished children showed poor performance on higher cortical functions like fluency, attention, working memory, visual perception, comprehension, learning and memory. These findings are supported by another study on Indian malnourished children, which reported memory impairments in undernourished children and spared fine motor coordination [22]. The malnourished children perform poor on novel tasks that require greater cognitive flexibility, like tests of executive functions.

Malnutrition and Cognitive Development

Malnutrition is known to have a detrimental effect on cognitive development. A few studies including the ones on Indian population have reported the influence of malnutrition on cognitive development. In one of the studies, 1336 children in the age range of 6-8 years Piagetian tasks covering the mental process of a concrete operational period were administered to examine cognitive development [23]. Weschler intelligence scale for Children was used to assess the intelligence of each child. The percentage of malnourished children in the preoperational stage, which is the first stage of cognitive development, was significantly higher as that of well-nourished children. A higher percentage of children in the other group were in concrete operation stage, which is the third stage of cognitive development. Performance on all the tasks was affected by under-nutrition. Nutrition was the only factor weakly associated with the poor performance of the children. Nutrition affected performance on conservation tasks more as compared to other tasks indicating poor verbal reasoning and comprehension. Information was also collected regarding the parental education and occupation. Environmental factors such as socio-economic status, caste, psychosocial stimulation and home environment were not found to be related to the detrimental effects of malnutrition.

In one of our studies discussed in the previous section, we have also found that development of cognitive functions is not only determined by age dependent effects but is also determined by the nutritional status. We studied effects of malnutrition with respect to stunting on cognitive development in children between 5-10 years of age. We did not find effect of age in isolation of the effect of nutrition.

Age related improvement in different cognitive functions was observed in adequately nourished children but not in malnourished children. However, rate of age related improvement might not uniformly be poor for all cognitive functions as we also found that the rate of improvement with age was not affected on certain functions like selective attention and verbal fluency in malnourished children (See Figures 1 & 2). However, working memory, design fluency, visuospatial relationships, learning, and memory showed slowing in terms of age related improvement in malnourished children. Motor speed and coordination were not affected (See Figures 2, 3 & 4). Most of the cognitive functions like fluency, working memory, visuo-spatial functions, comprehension, and memory have shown a very slow rate of improvement with age from early to middle childhood.

The rate of cognitive development was found to be different for different cognitive functions. Certain cognitive functions did not show regular age related changes whereas the changes could be observed on certain cognitive functions though not at the same level as in adequately nourished children.

Malnutrition affects brain growth and development and hence future behavioral outcomes [24]. School-age children who suffered from early childhood malnutrition have generally been found to have poorer IQ levels, cognitive function, school achievement and greater behavioral problems than matched controls and, to a lesser extent, siblings. The disadvantages last at least until adolescence. There is no consistent evidence of a specific cognitive deficit [25]. The functional integrity of specific cognitive processes is less clear. The only cognitive processes for which enduring cognitive changes were demonstrated in rehabilitated animals—outside of effects mediated by these affective changes—are cognitive flexibility and, possibly, susceptibility to proactive interference. Stunting in early childhood is common in developing countries and is associated with poorer cognition and school achievement in later childhood [26]. Deficits in children's scores have been reported to be smaller at age 11 years than at age 8 years in a longitudinal study on malnourished children stunted children suggesting that adverse effects may decline over time [27]. Adverse effects of malnutrition particularly stunting may decline with age only for certain cognitive functions but the rate of development for higher cognitive functions could be severely affected during the childhood years. The adverse effects of malnutrition (stunting) on cognitive development might be related to the delayed structural and functional maturation of the developing brain.

Summary and Conclusion

Malnutrition affects the rate of development of cognitive functions. The pattern of such effects could differ across cognitive functions. Chronic protein energy malnutrition affects the cognitive development during childhood years rather than only resulting in an overall cognitive impairment. Rate of development of executive functions, visuospatial functions and memory is more severely affected by protein energy malnutrition. It appears that certain cognitive functions could suffer from a more permanent deficit rather than just being a delay in development. Longitudinal studies on the effect of malnutrition on cognitive development would explain the pattern of developmental delay.

(Bhoomika R Kar is associated with Centre of Behavioural and Cognitive Sciences, University of Allahabad, Allahabad, 211001, UP, India.

Shobini L Rao and B A Chandramouli are associated with National Institute of Mental Health and Neurosciences, Hosur Road, Bangalore, Karnataka, India.)

References

[1] Udani PM: Protein Energy Malnutrition. Brain and various facets of child development. *Indian Journal of Pediatrics* 1992, 59: 165-186.

[2] Upadhyaya SK, Saran A, Agarwal DK, Singh MP, Agarwal KN: Growth and Behaviour Development in rural infants in relation to malnutrition and environment. *Indian Pediatrics* 1992, 29: 595-606.

[3] Upadhyaya SK, Agarwal KN, Agarwal DK: Influence of malnutrition on social maturity, visual motor coordination and memory in rural school children. *Indian Journal of Medical Research* 1989, 90: 320-327

[4] Upadhyay SK, Agarwal DK, Agarwal KN: Influence of malnutrition on intellectual development. *Indian Journal of Medical Research* 1989, 90: 430-441.

[5] Huttenlocher PR. Morphometric study of human cerebral cortex development. *Neuropsychologia,* 1990, 28: 517-527.

[6] Sowell ER, Trauner D A, Gamst A, Jernigan TL. Development of cortical and subcortical brain structures in childhood and adolescence: a structural MRI study. *Developmental Medicine and Child Neurology,* 2002, 44: 4-16.

[7] Spreen O, Risser AH, Edgell D. *Developmental neuropsychology* 1995, (pp. 3-77). New York: Oxford University Press.

[8] Thompson PM et al. Growth patterns in the developing brain detected by using continuum-mechanical tensor maps. *Nature,* 2000, 404: 190–193.

[9] Gogtay N, Giedd JN, Lusk L, Hayashi KM, Greenstein D, Vaituzis AC, Nugent TF 3rd, Herman DH, Clasen LS, Toga AW, Rapoport JL, Thompson PM. Dynamic mapping of human cortical development during childhood through early adulthood. *Proceedings of National Academy of Science, U.S.A.,* 2004, 101: 8174-8179.

[10] Sowell ER, Thompson PM, Leonard CM, Welcome SE, Kan E, Toga AW. Longitudinal mapping of cortical thickness and brain growth in normal children. *Journal of Neuroscience,* 2004, 24: 8223-8231

[11] Reuda MR, Rothbart MK, McCandliss BD, Saccommano L, Posner MI. Training, maturation and genetic influences on development of executive functions. *Proceedings of National Academy of Sciences,* 2005, 102: 14932-14936.

[12] Fuster JM. *The Prefrontal Cortex.* 1997, New York: Raven Press.

[13] Korkman M, Kemp SL, Kirk U. Effects of age on neurocognitive measures of children ages 5-12 years: A cross-sectional study on 800 children from the United States. *Developmental Neuropsychology,* 2001, 20: 331-354.

[14] Rebok GW, Smith CB, Pascualvaca DM, Mirsky AF, Anthony BJ, Kellam SG. *Child Neuropsychology,* 1997, 3: 28-46.

[15] Waber DP, De Moor C, Forbes PW, Almli CR, Botterson KN, Leonard G et al. The NIH MRI study of normal brain development: Performance of a population based sample of healthy children aged 6-18 years on a neuropsychological battery. *Journal of International Neuropsychological Society,* 2007, 13: 1-18.

[16] Levitsky DA, Strupp BJ. Malnutrition and the brain: changing concepts, changing concerns. *The Journal of Nutrition,* 1995, Suppl: 2212S-2220S.

[17] Posner MI, Petersen SE, Fox PT, Raichle ME: Localization of cognitive functions in the human brain. *Science,* 1988, 240: 1627-1631.

[18] Kar BR, Rao SL, Chandramouli BA. Cognitive development in children with chronic protein energy malnutrition. *Behavioural and Brain Functions,* 2008, *4:* 31.

[19] Raven J, Raven JC, Court JH. *Colored Progressive Matrices.* Oxford: Oxford Psychologists Press; 1998.

[20] Rutter MA. Children's Behaviour Questionnaire for completion by teachers: Preliminary findings. *Journal of Child Psychology and Psychiatry* 1967, 8: 1-11.

[21] Kar BR, Rao SL, Chandramouli BA, Thennarasu K. *NIMHANS Neuropsychological Battery for Children-Manual.* Bangalore: NIMHANS publication division; 2004.

[22] Agarwal KN, Agarwal DK, Upadhyay SK: Impact of chronic undernutrition on higher mental functions in Indian boys aged 10-12 years. *Acta Paediatrica* 1995, 84: 1357-61.

[23] Agarwal DK, Upadhyay SK, Agarwal KN. Influence of Malnutrition on Cognitive Development Assessed by Piagetian Tasks. Acta Pædiatrica, 1989, 78: 115 – 122.

[24] Gorman KS. Malnutrition and cognitive development: evidence from experimental/ quasiexperimental studies among the mild-moderately malnourished. *Journal of Nutrition* 1995, 125: 2239S-2244S.

[25] Grantham-McGregor S. A review of studies of the effect of severe malnutrition on mental development. *Journal of Nutrition Supplement*, 1995, 125: S2333–S2238.

[26] Chang SM, Walker SP, Grantham-McGregor S, Powell CA. Early childhood stunting and later behaviour and school achievement. *Journal of Child Psychology and Psychiatry*, 2002, 43: 775-783.

[27] Mendez M A, Adair LS. Severity and timing of stunting in the first two years of life affect performance on cognitive tests in late childhood. *Journal of Nutrition*, 1999, 129: 1555-1562.

Figure 1: Age Related Comparisons between Adequately Nourished and Malnourished Children on Selective Attention

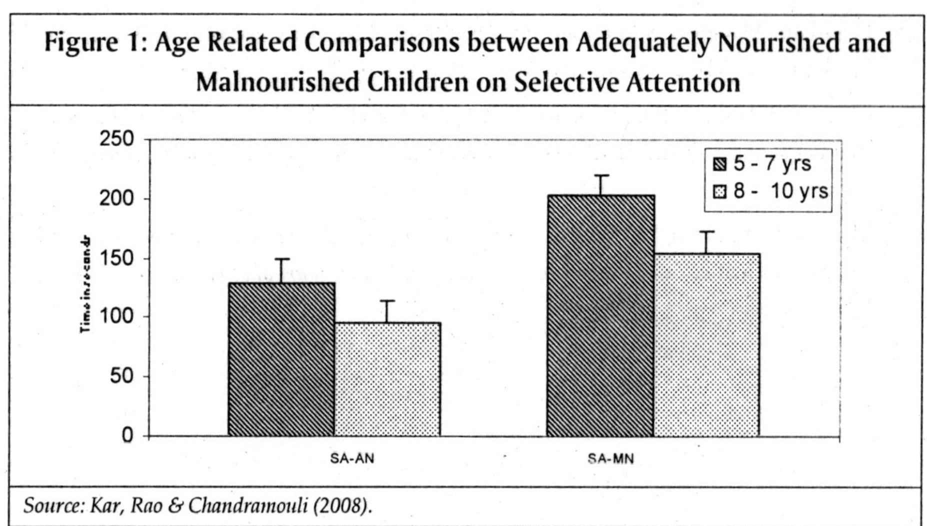

Source: Kar, Rao & Chandramouli (2008).

Figure 2: Age Related Comparisons between Adequately Nourished and Malnourished Children on Fluency and Working Memory

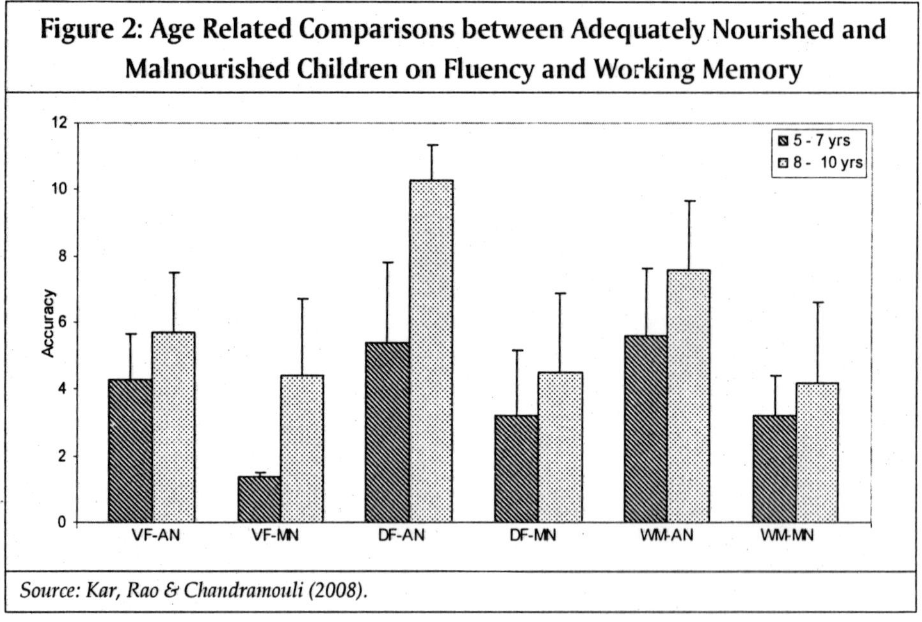

Source: Kar, Rao & Chandramouli (2008).

Figure 3: Age Related Comparisons between Adequately Nourished and Malnourished Children on Visuospatial Functions

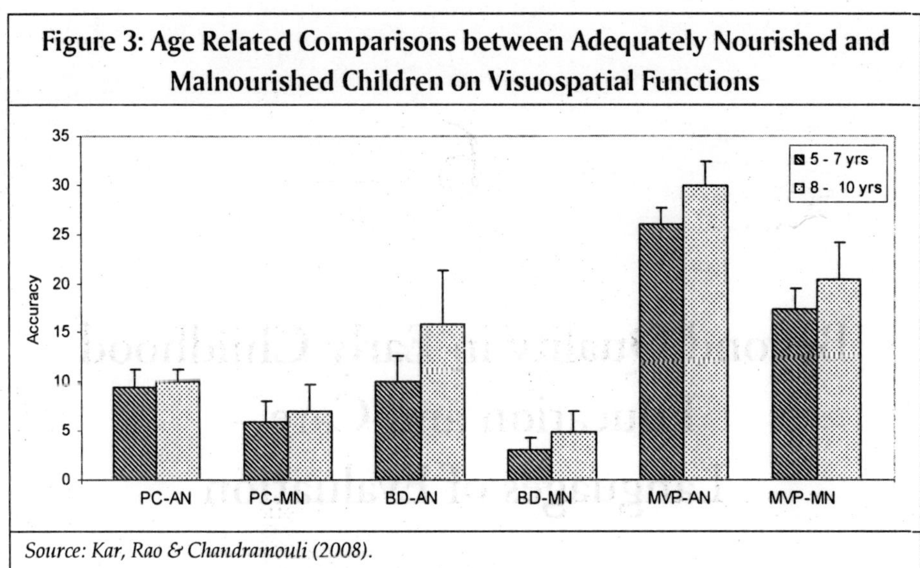

Source: Kar, Rao & Chandramouli (2008).

Figure 4: Age Related Comparisons between Adequately Nourished and Malnourished Children on Verbal and Visual Memory

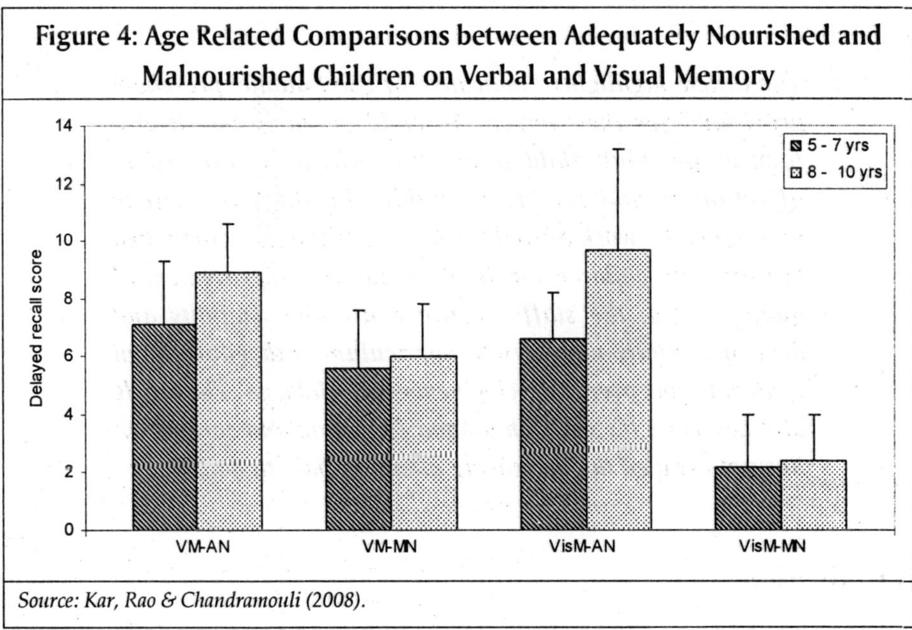

Source: Kar, Rao & Chandramouli (2008).

6

Beyond Quality in Early Childhood Education and Care – Languages of Evaluation

Peter Moss and Gunilla Dahlberg

The article highlights "indicative of good quality preschool provision" for their impact on child development. It also focuses on adult-child interaction which is responsive, affectionate and readily available. Further, the article highlights the work of well trained staffs that are committed to work with children for development and improvement of quality. Also, the staffs ensure continuity, stability and developmentally appropriate curriculum with educational content for the overall development of the children. The article also describes the early childhood education and care which has not escaped the increasing attention paid to quality.

Introduction

The problems which the managerial state is intended to resolve derive from contradictions and conflicts in the political, economic and social realms. But what we have seen is the managerialisation of these contradictions; they are redefined as

Source: CESifo DICE Report 2/2008 (www.cesifo-group.de) © CESifo, Munich. Reprinted with permission.

"problems to be managed". Terms such as "efficiency" and "effectiveness", "performance" and "quality" depoliticise a series of social issues (Whose efficiency? Effectiveness for whom?) and thus displace real political and policy choices into a series of managerial imperatives. (Clarke, 1998, p. 179)

We live in an age of quality. Every product and service must offer quality; every consumer wants to have it. In this historical context, quality has become reified, treated as if it was an essential attribute of services or products that gives them value, assumed to be natural and neutral. The problem with quality, from this perspective, is its management. How can quality be discovered, measured, assured and improved? What goals to be achieved by technical means will enhance performance and increase value?

Early childhood education and care has not escaped the increasing attention paid to quality; research and policy have become increasingly devoted to the subject. 'Quality' is generally understood as an attribute of services for young children that ensures the efficient production of predefined, normative outcomes, typically developmental or simple learning goals. Presence of quality is usually evaluated *vis-à-vis* expert-derived criteria, associated in research with achieving these outcomes. A recent report from a UK government agency, for example, commissioned a research review that identified seven factors "indicative of good quality pre-school provision" for their impact on child development: adult-child interaction that is responsive, affectionate and readily available; well-trained staff who are committed to their work with children; facilities that are safe and sanitary and accessible to parents; ratios and group sizes that allow staff to interact appropriately with children; supervision that maintains consistency; staff development that ensures continuity, stability and the improvement of quality; and a developmentally appropriate curriculum with educational content (National Audit Office, 2004, p. 39).

Nearly ten years ago, together with Alan Pence, we published a book, Beyond Quality in Early Childhood Education and Care (Dahlberg, Moss & Pence, 1999), that addressed an emerging and very different problem of quality, a problem not with the management of quality but with the very concept itself. It relativised quality, arguing that it was one way of talking about and practising evaluation, that quality was neither natural nor neutral, and was not therefore to be taken for granted. It was,

mindset for understanding the world and our position in it. In the case of quality, the progenitor paradigm is modernity – or, to be more precise, a particular paradigm of modernity, the paradigm of regulatory modernity (Hardt & Negri, 2001; Santos, 1998; Toulmin, 1990). The concept of quality is inscribed with the values and assumptions of that paradigm, some of which have been already mentioned: for example, the value given to certainty and mastery, linearity and predetermined outcomes, objectivity and universality. Believing in objectivity and the ability of science to reveal the true nature of a real world, modernity cannot recognise that it is a paradigm, a particular way of understanding the world produced within a particular historical and cultural context. It is unable to see itself as offering just one perspective, one way of thinking and practising.

Our conclusion in Beyond Quality is that quality is a child of its time and place, the product of particular nature and nurture. As such, the concept of quality:

> *cannot be conceptualized to accommodate complexity, values, diversity, subjectivity, multiple perspectives, and other features of a world understood to be both uncertain and diverse. The "problem with quality" cannot be addressed by struggling to reconstruct the concept in ways it was never intended to go. (Dahlberg, Moss & Pence, 2007, p. 105)*

Quality is a language of evaluation that fails to recognise a multilingual world and, in so doing, denies the possibility of other languages. And as Clarke describes in the quotation with which we begin the article, 'quality' is part of a process of depoliticisation that displaces "real political and policy choices into a series of managerial imperatives" – substituting managerial methods for democratic deliberation.

Meaning Making

Beyond Quality explores an other language of evaluation, meaning making, recognising that there may well be many others. The language of quality can be summed up as ending in a statement of fact: "it speaks of universal expert-derived norms and of criteria for measuring the achievement of these norms, quality being a measurement (often expressed as a number) of the extent to which services or practices conform to these norms" (Dahlberg, Moss & Pence, 2007, p. viii). Meaning making, by contrast, speaks of "evaluation as a democratic process of interpretation, a process that involves making practice visible and thus subject to reflection, dialogue and argumentation, leading to a judgement of value, contextualised and provisional because it is always subject to contestation" (p. ix).

Meaning making is evaluation as a participatory process of interpretation and judgement, made within a recognised context and in relation to certain critical questions: for example, what is our image of the child? what do we want for our children? what is education and care? It values subjectivity (or rather, 'rigorous subjectivity' (Lather 1991), uncertainty, provisionality, contextuality, dialogue and democracy. It assumes a participant who makes – in relation with others – a contextualised, subjective and rigorous judgement of value. It foregrounds, therefore, democratic political practice, the exercise of collective deliberation.

Meaning making employs particular methods, suited to its democratic political practice, in particular pedagogical documentation, a tool for participatory evaluation. Pedagogical documentation has its origins in the innovative and, today, world-famous municipal early childhood services in the Northern Italian city of Reggio Emilia (for further reading on Reggio Emilia and pedagogical documentation, see Dahlberg & Moss, 2005; Dahlberg, Moss & Pence, 2007; Giudici, Rinaldi & Krechevsky, 2001; Rinaldi, 2006). It requires, first of all, making practice visible through many forms of documentation: written or recorded notes, the work produced by children, photographs or videos, the possibilities are numerous. Then it requires a collective and democratic process of interpretation, critique and evaluation, involving dialogue and argumentation, listening and reflection, from which understandings are deepened and judgements co-constructed.

Its origins owe much to Loris Malaguzzi, one of the twentieth century's great pedagogical thinkers and practitioners and the first director of Reggio's municipal early childhood services. Documentation represents an extraordinary tool for dialogue, for exchange, for sharing. For Malaguzzi, it means the possibility to discuss and dialogue " 'everything with everyone' (teachers, auxiliary staff, cooks, families, administrators and citizens)...[S]haring opinions by means of documentation presupposes being able to discuss real, concrete things – not just theories or words, about which it is possible to reach easy and naïve agreement" (Hoyuelos, 2004, p. 7).

This concreteness of pedagogical documentation is critical. Measures of 'quality' involve looking for what has been predefined, discarding what does not figure in the template; it involves the decontextualised application of abstract criteria, reducing the complexity and concreteness of environment and practice to scores or boxes to tick; it strives for agreement and the elimination of different perspectives; it assumes the autonomous and objective (adult) observer. Above all, 'quality' offers consumers information about a product, for 'quality' is a language of evaluation suited to a particular understanding of early childhood (or other) services: as suppliers of commodities on the market to parent consumers.

Meaning making through documentation involves contextualised interpretations of actual practices and actual environments. It assumes that citizens participate with other citizens in the exercise of a public responsibility. This language of evaluation understands early childhood services as public forums and collective workshops, places of encounter for citizens young and old, with the potential for an infinite range of possibilities cultural, linguistic, social, aesthetic, ethical, political and economic – some expected and predetermined, but many that are not.

'Meaning making' therefore is generated from within a different discourse about democracy in general and early childhood in particular, a discourse which has a very different understanding than that of the managerial (and neo-liberal) discourse producing 'quality'. The discourse that generates meaning making also arises from a different paradigm which might be termed 'postfoundationalism', encompassing a variety of perspectives – for example, postmodernisms, poststructuralisms and postcolonialisms. This paradigm challenges the basic tenets, or foundations, of the paradigm of regulatory modernity: the possibility of objective, stable and value-free knowledge, universal laws, escaping context; the transparency and neutrality of language; linear progress ending in closure; dualistic – either/or – ways of thinking and relating to the world. It values what regulatory modernity finds problematic: complexity and multiplicity, subjectivity and context, provisionality and uncertainty. Post-foundationalism recognises that any phenomenon – early childhood education and care, for example – has multiple meanings, that any knowledge is perspectival, and that all experience is subject to interpretation.

Today, increasing numbers of scholars and practitioners in the early childhood field, across many countries, are working with postfoundational thinking and their theories and concepts have begun to influence practice and research. As the American early childhood researcher Joseph Tobin (2008) has noted, many scholars today "have drawn heavily on French social and philosophical theory (Foucault, Bourdieu, de Certeau, Althusser, Deleuze and Guattari) as well as feminist, queer, post-colonial theory to develop critical perspectives on dominant practice" (p. 23, original English version). In the series that we edit, Contesting Early Childhood, books published or in preparation draw heavily not only on the work of Foucault, but also of Derrida, Levinas, Delueze, Guattari and Bakhtin (Dahlberg & Moss, 2005; MacNaughton, 2006; Ermiston, 2007; Borgnon forthcoming; Lenz Taguchi in preparation). With their provocative perspectives and understandings, such work is introducing into the field of early childhood new thought, diverse forms of knowledge, and (literal and metaphorical) multilingualism.

Living in a Multi-lingual World

One of the dilemmas of trying to de-naturalise the language of quality – so that 'quality' can no longer be taken for granted as a neutral concept devoid of values or assumptions – and to differentiate it from another language, such as meaning making, is that the process may set up binary oppositions. The impression may be given that you must either go with quality or with meaning making, that it is a matter of either/or. But this has not been our intention; we argue for a multi-lingual world, where there is a continuing place for both – and other – languages of evaluation and, more broadly, for early childhood work to adopt different perspectives based on different paradigmatic positions.

We are more aware today than when we wrote Beyond Quality that the choices we make require far more than simply stating a preference. Working with the language of meaning making is difficult. It requires, or at least is greatly facilitated by, certain conditions: commitment to particular values, such as uncertainty, subjectivity, democracy; creativity, curiosity and a desire to experiment and border cross; a reflective, research-oriented and socially valued workforce; and sustained support from critical friends (for example, the pedagogistas or pedagogical coordinators in Reggio Emilia, who work closely and deeply with a small number of centres), networks of services, policy makers and politicians. Such conditions, we agree, are not widespread; and where they are lacking, it may be necessary to use the language of quality, which is easier to learn and speak, and requires the capacity to follow instructions and apply techniques correctly.

The decision to work with quality should, however, be viewed as a political choice made in a particular temporal and spatial context. The choice should be accompanied by the recognition that alternatives exist and by a view about future directions. Quality may be the right choice to make here and now, but is it the language of choice for 10 or 15 years hence? If yes, then what is the rationale for this stasis? And what are the dangers of staying with a language that is so strongly related to criteria and standards, that is so powerfully normalising and regulatory, that results in exclusion and lack of diversity? If no and if the intention is to learn and speak another language over time, or to become multi-lingual, then what conditions need putting in place, how will the transition be achieved? Will it be a general top-down change or will it be led by individual centres or networks of centres choosing to take up meaning making (or some other language of evaluation)? What norms and criteria will remain, even after these changes, since we think it is likely that even in the most decentralised and experimental system there will remain some normative framework, setting down some common values, principles, objectives and entitlements?

The recognition of different perspectives and a reluctance to limit possibilities by setting up either/or choices does not mean accepting uncritical relativism. Respecting other perspectives and positions does not free any of us from our responsibility to make a choice (for a fuller discussion of this issue, see Dahlberg & Moss, 2005). Thus, other perspectives and positions, the different languages of evaluation, are not a problem. What does present a problem is when others take a position as if no choice was involved, as if their position was the only one. So while we defend the right to adopt different perspectives and languages, we do so with an important proviso: that "all those engaged with early childhood and early childhood institutions recognise that there are different perspectives, that the work we do (whether as practitioners or parents or policy makers or researchers) always takes a particular perspective – and that therefore choices – or judgements of value – are always being made from which flow enormous implications in terms of theory and practice" (Dahlberg, Moss & Pence, 2007, p. 119).

Unfortunately, the acknowledgement of different perspectives is uncommon both among researchers and policy makers. Journal articles in the early childhood field frequently show no recognition of the authors' position with respect to paradigm and discourse, and its implications for defining questions in research and evaluation, the choice of methods and the interpretation of data. Although today there is a sort of standard policy document, produced by governments and international organisations, which offers a predictable rationale and prescription for early childhood education and care and draws on the same much-quoted research, it does not provide so much as one critical question or recognition that there may be different perspectives and views.

Not only do these documents make dull and repetitive reading. They stifle democracy. Political and ethical choices are replaced by a search for technical specifications. The current expansion of early childhood education and care provides, potentially, many benefits and possibilities for children, parents and wider society. But as Foucault enjoins us to remember, 'everything is dangerous, but not always bad', and expansion brings with it major risks, not least of which is increasing regulation and normalisation, what Nikolas Rose (1999) terms 'governing the soul'.

If these risks are to be reduced and the potential benefits realised, societies need to put technical and managerial practice in its place, as subservient to democratic political and ethical practice, and to open themselves to diversity and experimentation.

(Peter Moss is associated with Institute of Education, University of London.

Gunilla Dahlberg is associated with Stockholm Institute of Education, Sweden.)

References

Balaguer, I., Mestres, J., & Penn, H. (1992). Quality in services for young children. Brussels: European Commission Equal Opportunities Unit.

Borgnon, L. (in press). Movement and experimentation in young children's learning. London: Routledge.

Clarke, J. (1998). Thriving on Chaos? Managerialisation and Social Welfare. In J. Carter (Ed.), Postmodernity and the fragmentation of welfare (pp. 171-186). London: Routledge.

Dahlberg, G., Lundgren, U. P., & Åsén, G. (1991), Att utvärdera barnomsorg (To evaluate early childhood care and education). Stockholm: HLS Förlag.

Dahlberg, G., & Moss, P. (2005). Ethics and politics in early childhood education. London: Routledge Falmer.

Dahlberg, G., Moss, P., & Pence, A. (1999). Beyond quality in early childhood education and care: Postmodern perspectives (1st Ed.). London: Falmer Press.

Dahlberg, G., Moss, P., & Pence, A. (2007). Beyond quality in early childhood education and care: Languages of evaluation (2nd Ed.). London: Falmer Press.

Ermiston, B. (2007). Forming ethical identities in early childhood play. London: Routledge. European Commission Childcare Network (1996). Quality targets in services for young children. Brussels: European Commission Equal Opportunities Unit.

Evans, J. (1994). Quality in ECCD: Everyone's concern. Coordinators' Notebook, 15, 1-32.

Farquhar, S. (1993). Breaking new ground in the study of quality. Paper presented at the NZARE annual conference, Hamilton, New Zealand.

Giudici, C., Rinaldi, C., & Krechevsky, M. (Eds.) (2001). Making learning visible: Children as individual and group learners. Cambridge, MASS. & Reggio Emilia: Project Zero & Reggio Children.

Hardt, M., & Negri, A. (2001). Empire. Cambridge, MASS: Harvard University Press.

Hoyuelos, A. (2004). A pedagogy of transgression. Children in Europe, 6, 6-7.

Lather, P. (1991). Getting smart: Feminist research and pedagogy with/in the postmodern. London: Routledge.

MacNaughton, G. (2005). Doing Foucault in early childhood studies: Applying poststructural ideas. London: Routledge Falmer.

Moss, P. & Pence, A. (Eds.) (1994). Valuing quality in early childhood services. London: Paul Chapman Publishing.

Munton, A., Mooney, A. & Rowland, L. (1995). Deconstructing quality: A conceptual framework for the new paradigm in day care provision for the under eights. Early Childhood Development and Care, 114, 11-23.

National Audit Office (2004). Early years: Progress in developing high quality childcare and early education accessible to all. London: The Stationery Office.

Pascal, C., Bertram, A., & Ramsden, F. (1994). The effective early learning research project: The quality, evaluation and development process. Worcester, UK: Worcester College of Higher Education.

Pence, A. (1992). Quality care: Thoughts on r/rulers. Paper presented at a workshop on Defining and Assessing Quality, Seville, Spain.

Power, M. (1997). The audit society. Oxford: Oxford University Press.

Rose, N. (1999). Powers of freedom: Reframing political thought. Cambridge: Cambridge University Press.

Santos, B. de S. (1995). Towards a new common sense: Law, science and politics in the paradigmatic transition. London: Routledge.

Santos, B. de S. (2004). Interview with Boaventura de Sousa Santos. Globalisation, Societies and Education, 2(2), 147-60.

Tobin, J. (2008), Rôle de la théorie dans le mouvement reconceptualiser l'éducation de la petite enfance (The role of theory in the reconceptualising early childhood education movement). in G. Brougère, & M. Vandenbroeck (Eds.), Repenser l'éducation des jeunes enfants (pp. 23-52). Bruxelles: Peter Lang.

Toulmin, S. (1990), Cosmopolis: The hidden agenda of modernity. Chicago: University of Chicago Press.

Williams, P. (1994). Making sense of quality: A review of approaches to quality in early childhood services. London: National Children's Bureau.

Woodhead, M. (1996). In search of the rainbow: Pathways to quality in large scale programmes for young disadvantaged children. The Hague: Bernard van Leer Foundation.

7

Parenting and Responsibility
Holding Parents Accountable for Children's Antisocial Practices

E A Uwe, P N Asuquo and E E Ekuri

Proper nurturing of children is the primary responsibility of parents. Parents have inescapable responsibilities when bringing up their children. These responsibilities are automatically conferred on the parents of the child right from the child's birth. They are expected to guide and modify the behaviour of their child to conform with the acceptable behaviours in the society as well as participate in activities aimed at preventing crime or disorder being committed by their children. Ironically, some parents have failed in these roles and functions. They adopt too much permissive and laissez-faire parenting styles that inadvertently make their children vulnerable to anti-social behaviours. This paper focuses on parents as the catalysts for children's behaviour. The rationale for children's anti-social behaviours are highlighted as well as some of the corrupt behaviours parents exhibit. The root causes of these behaviours are brought to the limelight and suggestions proffered for improving the task of parenting.

Source: www.krepublishers.com, Journal of Human Ecology Vol. 24, Issue 1, pp. 51-57, September 2008.

Introduction

Youth are our expected future leaders. In a society where these would be future leaders are engaged in crimes, violence, and other delinquent and corrupt behaviours, there can never be peace, progress and sustainable development. Peace is an important phenomenon, a condition the nation, the world and every individual need. In the absence of peace there is the possibility of instability, insecurity, burglary, thugery, assault, rape, street ganging, drug peddling and abuse, and other vices.

In our contemporary Nigerian setting, the authors observed that a lot of people exhibit dishonest behaviours without any fear of apprehension. Some of these behaviours include taking part in bank fraud, taking loans from banks without adequate collateral, demanding bribe before appointment is offered to prospective applicants, money laundering, involvement in massif scale theft popularly known as '419' or Advanced Fee Fraud and getting bribe and setting culprits free from prison custody.

In the urban areas, the streets and residences are no longer safe, no matter how well fortified they may be. Streets-smart-boys, popularly known as "Area-boys" are found everywhere roaming the streets, harassing and extorting money from innocent people. The youth are involved in non-cultism, armed robbery, examination malpractices, assaults, rape, violence, substance abuse, alcoholism, certificate racketing and vandalism, to mention but a few. Sadly enough, children manifest some of these antisocial behaviours before they even start school.

These corrupt practices have dominated the social landscape of the nation for decades. They have been so prevalent in both low and high places that it has necessitated the establishment of some structures by the Federal Government, such as the Tribunal for Corrupt Practices (TCP), Code of Conduct Bureau (CCB). Nigerian Drug Law Enforcement Agency (NDLEA), Anti-Trade Malpractice Commission (AMC), Economic and Financial Crimes Commission (EFCC), Independent Corrupt Practice Commission (ICPC) and others to check such negative behaviours.

This prevailing atmosphere has given rise to some pondering questions as to what could have been the possible root causes of children, youth and even adults involvement in antisocial behaviours. Could parents, who are expected to be the custodians of appropriate behaviour in children be held accountable for such behaviours as a result of their laxity and failure in carrying out their parental responsibilities? Do they in one way or the other contribute to their children's involvement in anti-social practices?

Parenting in the Nigerian context entails the nurturing relationship between the parents (or parent in the case of single parents) and the child. In this relationship the parents have the responsibility and obligation to meet the needs of the child, as well as teach the child ethical and spiritual principles of the society. The parents are expected to pass on the societal values, such as, respect for others, self-control, goodness, altruism, truth, fairness and honesty.

The family in which parents are the leaders is a great socialization agent. It is the first social setting that a child experiences in life. Within this social setting, the child begins his socialization process. The family is therefore involved in molding the individual behaviour from the formative stage. Once the family fails in its obligations, the entire society stands to suffer the consequences.

Unfortunately, some parents who are at the head of this socialization unit expose their children to antisocial behaviours. Some of them use their children in planting and/or peddling Indian hemp and other dangerous substances. Some purchase fake certificates for their children to gain admission into higher institutions of learning and some even pay huge sums of money to their children's teachers/lecturers to alter their failed grades, etc.

Rationale for Children's Anti-Social Behaviour

Our children represent the future generation, and so, they must be properly molded for their future roles. The child's parents have the greatest part to play in this molding process as they are the first socializing agents to the child. Therefore, the type of training the parents give the child and the values they propagate will determine the future life style of the child. This is because once an attitude has been established concerning a certain behaviour, it becomes difficult to eradicate (Pierson and Thomas, 2002).

In Skinner's (1953) instrumental theory, also known as 'operant conditioning', he demonstrated that the environment has a much greater influence on learning and behaviour. This is mostly observed at the formative period of one's life. Environmental response to behaviour according to Skinner serves either to reinforce or eliminate learning and behaviour. According to Skinner, if a response is reinforced, it is more likely for that behaviour to re-occur. Therefore parents who reinforce antisocial behaviours in their children encourage such behaviour to reoccur. So, it is the responsibility of parents to always respond appropriately to their children's behaviour so that the obnoxious ones are eliminated, while the accepted ones are strengthened.

Nagin and Farrington (1992) also believe that the tendency to commit crime is established early in life, perhaps around the pre-school years, and this is the period that the home environment determines almost all that the child does or leaves undone for example, his actions and inactions. According to them once a child manifests an unwanted behaviour, he is likely to behave that way again when such conditions occur. This position is in line with Wilson and Herrnstein's (1985) theoretical assertion that there exists a positive association between past and future criminal behaviour. To them, the best predictor of crime is past criminal behaviour.

Sutherland (1973), in his theory of differential association, arrived at some principles related to delinquent behaviours. The first principle is that delinquent behaviour is learned. He argued that only sociological explanation could account for a person's involvement in delinquency. The second principle is that delinquent behaviour is learned, while communicating with others in intimate groups. Sutherland and Cressey (1978) in their investigation focused on the family or peer group as the most likely source of initiation into delinquent value and activities. The third principle according to Sutherland (1973) claims that learning process includes two different elements, techniques (how to commit offences) and attitudes or rationalization (how to justify the offences against self and others). The fourth principle states that rationalization and attitudes toward the law are learned from people whom we associate with and who hold attitudes that favour either obeying the laws or violating them. The fifth principle states that people who are more exposed to verbal signs and suggestions will break the law more than those who are obedient. Thus, parents who give the hint that it is acceptable to fight, cheat or lie may foster delinquent children. However, the sixth principle espoused by Sutherland is that the longer and earlier youth are exposed to a set of attitudes about delinquency, the more influenced they will be.

Bandura (1971) in his social learning theory stressed the potent influence of modelling on behaviour. He argued that behaviour is the joint product of the person and the environment. He acknowledges that people can alter their environment, which therefore turn round to alter their behaviour. In his view of behaviour change processes, Bandura places great prominence on observational learning and modelling. According to Bandura, practically all of the learning that people can acquire through their own direct experience could be acquired vicariously. This implies that such behaviour is acquired at second hand by observing someone else. Four processes influence observation of learning process in Bandura's view, namely: attention, retention, performance and motivation. People attend to the behaviour of a model and retain the modelled information, which is aided by imagery and verbal coding and then perform the act so modelled by putting the appropriate motor movement from the information gained. Motivation therefore, determines whether or not the person will deploy the behaviour so modelled.

Aggression is to a great extent a learned behavour (Bandura, 1973; Berkowitz, 1962; Eron, Walder and Leftkowitz, 1971). Morton (1987) argued that socio-culturally, delinquent children are frequently reared in homes that offer little understanding, affection, stability or moral clarity. Lotz (1979) in his study also found that person turn to crime because they were not given enough discipline when young. Monteleone (1996), Ekpo (1996) and Uwe and Obot (2000) in their view, argued that when parents fail to teach their children the necessary social skills for successful interaction in the world, such parents automatically leave the children vulnerable to learn inappropriate behaviours from those who would take advantage of them. This further assert that parents who themselves display antisocial behaviours commonly transmit such values, action and attitudes to their children.

Commenting on the cost of pathological gambling to families and friends, Awake (2002) reported that problems of gambling spread from parents to child, in that, children of compulsive gambling parents are likely to engage in delinquent behaviours, such as, smoking, drinking and using drugs. The children also have an increased risk of developing problems of pathological gambling themselves. Awake (2002) further reported a survey result in the United Kingdom, which found that, among adolescents who gamble, 46 percent stole from their family to support their habit.

Monteleon (1996) argued that corrupting could begin with rewarding the infants; encouraging violence towards peers; laughing at anti-social behaviours; and encouraging children to sell, deliver and use drugs. Single parenthood also play a part in the degenerative function of the family. Swadener (1990), Lubeck and Garrett (1990) and Ekpo (1996) opined that adolescents who terrorize people particularly in urban areas, do so because their single-parents households have failed in adequately teaching them the value of human life and decency.

Some parents are hostile, indifferent and rarely show affection to their children Uwe (1997). They neglect or beat their children, but rarely exercise consistent firm guidance. Some are so permissive that they do not care about what happens to their children, or what they do. Such parents according to Bandura and Walter (1959), and Glueck and Glueck (1960) produce delinquent children. Furthermore, in permissive homes, children get premature autonomy. They come and go as they wish. With such inconsistent parents, children become relatively confused as to the reactions they would get. As an example, coming home late one day, may result in scolding or beating, and coming late next day may be overlooked. Patterson (1980) affirmed that not only do parents of chronic delinquents not know how to parent effectively, but also many of them do not care. Wahua (2001) opined that some parents even rise to the children's defence and accuse others for picking on their children even when it is obvious that the children have committed the crime of which they are accused.

Some parents do not display proper role model for their children to emulate (Uwe 1997). They openly display anti-social behaviours before their children, for example offering and accepting bribes. Some parents who experienced abusive parenting from their parents continue to perpetuate these negative attitude thereby making their children become toughened and so the cycle goes on. In Ekanem's (2000) view, there are also parents who do not have time to talk with their children nor listen to them. Such children are left on their own and have no feelings of being wanted. They do not develop good sense of self-worth and positive self-concept. As a result of this neglect the children judge themselves as misfits with unbalanced personality.

Ekanem (2000) argued that parents who do not establish a clear consistent boundaries and limits for their children could be so permissive that children are left unguided as to what the acceptable behaviour should be. Such children according to her often put themselves into unwarranted problems even with law enforcement agents.

Parents as Perpetuators of Corrupt Behaviours

Children's welfare and rights have been a central concern of the United Nations since its inception in 1945. The United Nations Convention On the Rights of the Child (1991) acknowledges the primary role of the family and parents in the care and protection of children. According to the Convention, parents have the primary responsibility for the child's upbringing. Unfortunately, this primary function has degenerated and has not been achieved as expected. This degenerative symptom of the family has permeated the entire social fabric of the nation. Parents, instead of enhancing positive development in their children, knowingly or unknowingly encourage and reinforce children's anti-social behaviour.

Many sociologists, such as Sears *et al.* (1957), Patterson (1976), Whaler (1976), Atkeson and Forehand (1981), Monteleone (1996), assert that parent-child interaction is central in shaping and maintaining high level of either positive or negative behaviours. Monteleone (1996) argued that parents who ignore or reinforce delinquent behaviour are corrupt themselves. Patterson (1976) views a coercive family as breeding aggressive children. He opined that a coercive method of interpersonal control predominates in such families. According to him, this pattern of family interaction develops as a result of parental deficits in child management.

Parent's Contribution to Children's Anti-social Behaviours

Parents as leaders should be role models. Achebe (1998) asserts that people look up to their leaders as role models. They copy their actions, behaviour and even mannerisms. Achebe (1998: 37) stated therefore that "if a leader lacks discipline the effect is apt to spread automatically down to his followers". The implication is that, if parents as leaders to be emulated by their children exhibit negative behaviours, then the tendency will be that children, their followers will copy those behaviours.

Moneteleon (1996) asserts that some parents go to the extent of conveying approval of, or encourage their children's precocious interest in the areas of sexuality, aggression, violence and substance abuse. He enumerated some parental corrupt behaviours as follows:

- Allowing and/or forcing child to watch pornographic materials
- Teaching child sexually exploitative behaviours,
- Teaching child illegal activity,
- Knowingly allowing others to teach illegal activity to the child,
- Praising child for antisocial/illegal activity,
- Assisting child in delinquent behaviour,
- Failing to discipline child for delinquent behaviour,
- Teaching child that "bad is good and good is bad",
- Giving drugs or other contraband to child,
- Exposing child to harmful influences or situations,
- Using child as a spy, ally or confident in parents romantic relationships, marital or divorce problem (p. 129).

Other corrupt behaviours in parents observed by researchers such as Ekpo (1996), Isangedighi (1997), Okon (1997), Uwe (1997), Ekanem (2000), Eweniyi (2000), Obot (2000), Uwe et al. (2004) include:

- Sexual exploitation of children, for example encouraging prostitution by introducing teenage girls to "Sugar Daddies" for monetary gains;
- Master sleeping with his housemaid;
- Allowing children sleep on the same bed with adult family friends thereby encouraging assault and rape;
- Sending young children as forced or bonded servants in exchange of small loans or payment of debt thus encouraging child abuse;

- Involvement of children in planting and peddling Indian hemp and other substances;
- Involvement in human trafficking;
- Use of children in errands to purchase items such as cigarettes, drugs, alcohol including ogogoro (illicit gin);
- Encouraging the child to grow faster than his/her age, for example, perming a child's hair, using adult make-up on the child and allowing the child out with peers unknown to parents and without their permission;
- Failure to provide the necessary control, or role model for learning socialization and responsible behaviour;
- Ritualistic abuse of the child, for example, using a girl child as a maiden in the worship of water goddess;
- Involvement of children in gambling;
- Offering and accepting bribes even before the child;
- Purchasing fake certificate for child to gain admission into higher institution of learning;
- Paying lecturers and teachers to alter a child's failed scores;
- Misappropriation of public funds;
- Non-completion of contract transaction;
- Dishonesty in business dealings, for example, swearing falsely before the child to customers;
- Swindling in the name of religion;
- Encouraging school absence to enable the child go street hawking;
- Withdrawal of child prematurely from school for exploitative purposes;
- Verbal battering of the child;
- Impaired parenting; and
- Trafficking drug by hiding substances on an innocent infant's body.

Possible Causes of Parental Corrupt Behaviours

The causes of parental corrupt behaviour are complex, multiple and interactive. Decay and Travers (1996) opined that constitutionally more males than females commit crimes and that younger males than older males are involved in criminal behaviour. The also argue that developmentally broken families are more prone to crime than intact families.

Poverty is a leading possible cause of parental antisocial behaviours. In our Nigerian setting, having many children receives social approval and honour (Afuekwe 1992). Many parents end up breeding many children without the necessary resources to cater for them. They often hope that God would provide for their needs. With the austere economic situation in the nation, the dearth of employment and inflation, such parents have too many mouths to feed, more so as their young adult children continue to depend on them for their needs because of unemployment. Forced by their circumstances, such parents indulge themselves in antisocial activities in order to sustain the family.

Another important cause of parental corrupt behaviour is greed. The society is moving very fast in fashion and wealth because of globalization and information technology. Everyone wants to be like the Joneses, driving expensive cars and living in luxurious apartments. There is an axiom which says that "money is the root of all evil". Everybody wants to have it either by crook or crude way. Money has become a surrogate god to many and greed is a debilitating social sickness. Greed and lust for money drive many parents into crimes.

Some parents find it hard to revolutionize the way they were brought up (Monteleone 1996). They repeat the parenting cycle and pass on the type of parenting they received. Some are so permissive and non-challant. They are less interested in bringing up the child in the acceptable way. Moreover, attitude of Nigerians towards corrupting behaviour is appalling. Corrupt behaviours are sometimes regarded as normal and anybody who succeeds and gets away, feels he/she is intelligent afterall.

Recommendations for Improved Parenting Skills

There is the need to bring up children that are well-adjusted. To assist parents meet their responsibilities, the following strategies are recommended:

- Parents should display proper role model for children to emulate;
- They should show enough affection to their children.
- They should endeavour to stop perpetuating abusive parenting that they themselves went through.
- Parents should find time to talk with their children and also listen to them in order to get into their innermost feelings, thoughts and emotion and guide them properly.
- Children should be helped to develop the sense of self worth and positive self concept. This is because the way the child judges himself determines how balance his personality is.
- Clear consistent boundaries should be set for children. These help to guide children on the acceptable behaviour by parents.
- There should be regular monitory of what children do.
- Parents should create a secure environment where peace, love and harmony prevail.
- Lastly, priority should be given to spirituality. Parents should meditate on the scriptures, pray and worship together with their children.

Conclusion

Parents have some responsibilities which they can never escape from in as much as they bring children into this world. They are responsible for meeting the physical, social, emotional, psychological and spiritual needs of their children. Through proper socialization, they are expected to nurture the children and groom them, ready for launching them into the society. Unfortunately, some of these parents fail in these responsibilities and rather encourage some antisocial behaviours in their children. They openly exhibit those maladaptive behaviours for children to emulate and do not monitor what their children do. There is therefore the need to arrest this prevailing conditions if the country is to forge ahead in its sustainable development programmes. As future leaders it is imperative to 'catch' the youth when they are young. When children are well-adjusted and disciplined, the nation, the citizenry and the world at large will experience peace.

(E A Uwe, P N Asuquo and E E Ekuri, Department of Educational Foundations, University of Calabar, Calabar, Nigeria.)

References

Achebe, C.: *The Trouble with Nigeria.* Fourth Dimension Publishing Company, Enugu (1998).

Afuekwi, C. I.: *A philosophical inquiry into religious and Scoial life in Igbo land: Alor as a case study.* Associated Publishers and Consultants, Calabar: (1992).

Atkeson, B. M. and Forehand R. (1981). Conduct disorders. In: *Behaviour Assessment Of Childhood Disorders.* E. J. and I. O. Terdal (Eds.). Guilford, New York. (1981).

Awake: *What is Wrong with Gambling.* Watchtower Bible and Tract Society, New York July 22 (2002).

Bandura, A.: Psychotherapy based upon modelling principles. Pp. 653-708. In: *Handbook of Psychotherapy and Behaviour Change.* A. E. Bergin and S. L. Garfield (Eds.). Wiley, New York (1971).

Bandura, A. and Walters, R. H.: *Adolescent Aggression.* Ronald, New York (1959).

Berkowitz, L.: *Aggression: A Social Psychological Analysis.* McGraw-Hill, Boston (1962).

Decay, J. S. and Travers, J. F.: *Human Development Across the Life Span.* Boston: McGraw-Hill, Boston (1996).

Ekanem, T. F.: Parental care and child moral development. *UJOWACS. University of Uyo Journal of Women Academics,* **1(1)**: 157-163 (2000).

Ekpo, S.: *Juvenile Delinquency in Nigeria.* ABBNNY Educational Publishers, Uyo (1996).

Eron, L. O., Walder, I. O. and Leftkowitz, M. M.: *The Learning of Aggression in Children.* Little, Brown, Boston (1971).

Eweniyi, G. B.: Child Sexual Abuse and the Rights of the Nigerian Child. *The Counsellor.* 18(1): 166-172 (2000).

Glueck, S. and Glueck, E.: *Unraveling Juvenile delinquency.* Commonwealth Fund, New York (1960).

Isangedighi, A. J.: Youth on the margins: Indices of indiscipline behaviour. *Nigerian Journal of Educational Foundations,* 1(1): 18-20 (1997). Lotz, R.: Public anxiety about crime. *Pacific sociological Review.* 22: 241-254 (1979).

Lubeck, S. and Garrett, P.: The social construction of the "at risk" child. *Journal of Sociology of Education,* 11(3): 327-340 (1990).

Monteleone, J. A.: *Recognition of child abuse for the mandated.* Reporter, G. W. medical Publishing, St. Louis, Missiour (1996).

Morton, I.: Childhood aggression in the context of family Interactions. In: *Childhood Aggression and Violence.* D. Crowell, I. Evans, and C. Odonnell (Eds.). Plenum Press, New York New York: (1987).

Nagin, D. and Farrington, D.: The stability of criminal potential from childhood and adulthood. *Criminology,* 30: 235-260 (1992).

Obot, A. E.: Single Parenthood. In: *Marriage Counselling: Issues and Solutions.* E. A. Uwe and A. E. Obong (Eds.). Pyramid Publishers, Calabar (2000).

Okon, M. O.: Parental role in Behaviour Modification: Implication for Counselling. *The Calabar Counsellor,* 1(2): 138-145 (1997).

Patterson, G. R.: The aggressive child: Victim and architect of a cursive system. In: *Behaviour Modification and family.* L. G. Hamerlynck, L. C. Handy, and E. J. Masia (Eds.). Brunner/Mazel, New York (1976).

Patterson, G. R..: Children who steal. In: *Understanding Crime.* I. Hirschi, and M. Gottfredson (Eds.) Sage, Berverly Hills, Calif. (1980).

Pierson, J. and Thomas, M.: *Collins Dictionary: Social Work.* HarperCollins Publishers, Great Britain (2002).

Sears, R. R., Maccoby, E. E.; and Levin, H.: *Patterns of Child Rearing.* Harpey and Row, New York (1957). Skinner, B. F.: *Science and Human Behaviour.* The Free Press, New York (1953).

Sutherland, E. H.: *On Analyzing of Crime* University of Chicago Press, Chicago (1973).

Sutherland, E. H., and Cressey, D. R.: *Criminology.* Lippihcott, Philadelphia (1978).

Swadener, E. B.: Children and families "at risk": Etiology, Critique and alternative paradigms. *Educational Foundations,* 4(4): 17-39 (1990).

United Nations: *Convention on the Rights of the Child.* United Nations, New York (1991).

Uwe, E. A.: Parental Roles in Behaviour modification of youth. *The Calabar Counsellor* 1(1): 121-126 (1997).

Uwe, E. A. and Obot, A. E.: *Marriage Counselling: Issues and Solutions.* Pyramid Publishers, Calabar (2000).

Uwe, E. A., Ekuri, E. E. e. and Asuquo, P. N.: African Women and Vulnerability to HIV/AIDS: Implications on Female related Cultural Practices. *A Paper Presented at the Pan African Anthropological Association Conference,* Legon, Ghana August 2nd-6th (2004).

Wahua, T. A. T.: *Home Harmony:* Dalitt Publishing Company (2001).

Whaler, R. O.: Deviant child behaviour within the family: Develomental speculations and behaviour change strategies. In: *Handbood of Behaviour Modification.* H. Leitengerg (Ed.). Prentice-Hall, Englewood Cliffs, N. J. (1976).

Wilson, J. and Herrnstein, R.: *Crime and Human Nature.* Simon and Schuster, New York (1985).

Section II

Country Experiences

8

Intra-Urban and Intra-Rural Inequities in Child Health: Evidence from Sub-Saharan Africa

Jean-Christophe Fotso

Over the last few decades, sub-Saharan Africa has witnessed an urban population explosion despite poor macroeconomic performance, making it difficult for national and urban authorities to provide affordable housing, quality social services, or sufficient employment to the growing urban populations. Recent estimates indicate that about 42 percent of the urban population in most sub-Saharan African countries live in "life and health threatening" homes or neighborhoods. On the other hand, improvements in child survival have been very poor in sub-Saharan Africa, and progress in child nutritional well-being observed world wide continues to bypass many African countries and population subgroups. Against the foregoing backdrop, this paper seeks to revisit the urban advantage in health by examining differences across urban and rural areas in health inequalities. Specifically, its goal is to compare the magnitude of inequities in child malnutrition across urban and rural areas; and compare the intra-urban inequities with urban-rural differences.

We use recent Demographic and Health Surveys (DHS) data from 25 sub-Saharan African countries, with stunting malnutrition as the child health variable of interest. A wealth index variable is computed separately for urban and rural areas in each country and recoded in three categories labelled as poorest, middle and rich as the measure of child health. The poor-to-rich and rural-to-urban ratios of malnutrition are used as a proxies for inequities. Our results indicate that in all countries and areas (urban or rural), children from poorest households have greater risk of malnutrition compared to their counterparts in the most privileged households. More importantly, while malnutrition is, on average, higher in rural settings compared to urban areas, disparities between the poor and the rich are, to a large extent, higher in cities than in rural areas. The study also reveals that intra-urban inequities in child malnutrition are even larger than urban-rural differentials in malnutrition.

Overall, this study suggests that failing to appropriately target the growing sub-group of the urban poor and improve their living conditions and health status, policies and programs geared at improving children's welfare, including the MDGs, may not meet their national goals. In addition to improving the overall urban and national averages of health indicators, it is important to analyze, track and purposefully reduce health inequities, since progress towards the achievement of the health MDGs will not automatically benefit the underprivileged population sub-groups.

1. Introduction

Urbanization and Poverty in Sub-Saharan Africa

Over the last few decades, the world has witnessed an urban population explosion, with nearly forty-five per cent of the world's population living in urban areas in 2005.

The proportion is projected to exceed 50 per cent by 2007, thus making it the first time in history that the world has more urban than rural residents (United Nations, 2007). Within this general context, cities in sub-Saharan Africa have experienced the fastest population growth, and most of the future population growth in the region is expected to occur in urban areas. The region's urban population was about 20% in 1970, 35 percent in 2005, and is projected to near 50 percent by 2030 (World Bank, 2008). In terms of growth, while urban population in sub-Saharan Africa increased by an average of 4.7% annually between 1970 to 2005 (from 56.1 to 264.4 millions), the rural population only grew by 2.1% (from 236.9 to 486.9 millions). Figure 1 depicts the evolution of urban, rural and total sub-Saharan Africa's population from 1970, assuming a starting size of 100 (base 100 in 1970). The urban population increased nearly five-fold between 1970 and 2005 (from 100 to 471), and is projected to be about 11 times its 1970 size by 2030. Rural population only doubled between 1970 and 2005 (from 100 to 206) and is expected to reach less than three times its 1970 size by 2030.

Figure 1: Evoluation of Sub-Saharan African Urban, Rural and Total Population (1970-2030): Index base 100 in 1970

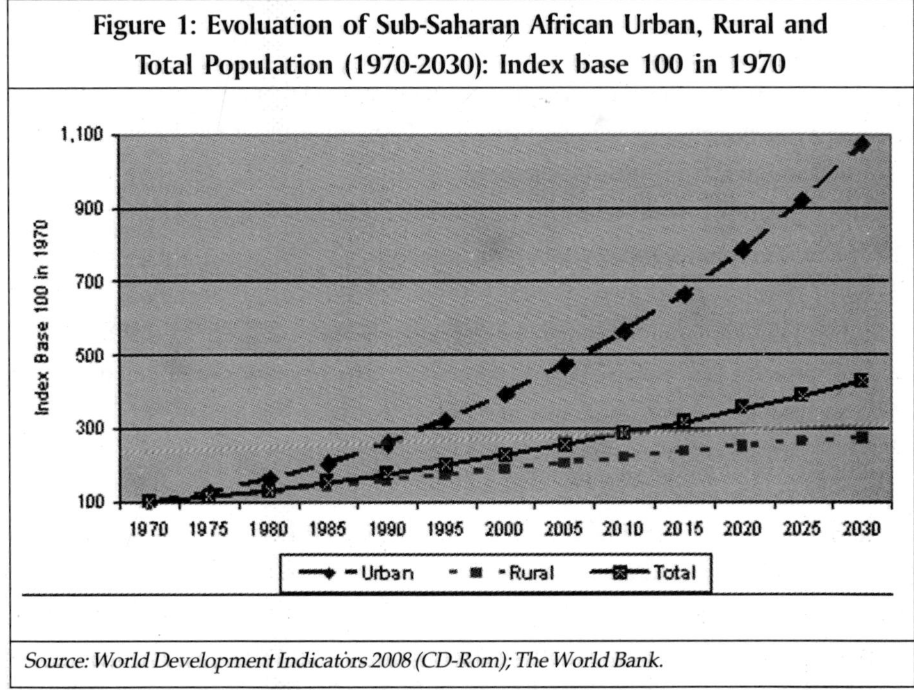

Source: World Development Indicators 2008 (CD-Rom); The World Bank.

Figure 2: Evolution of Sub-Saharan African urban population and per capita GDP (1975-2005): Index base 100 in 1975

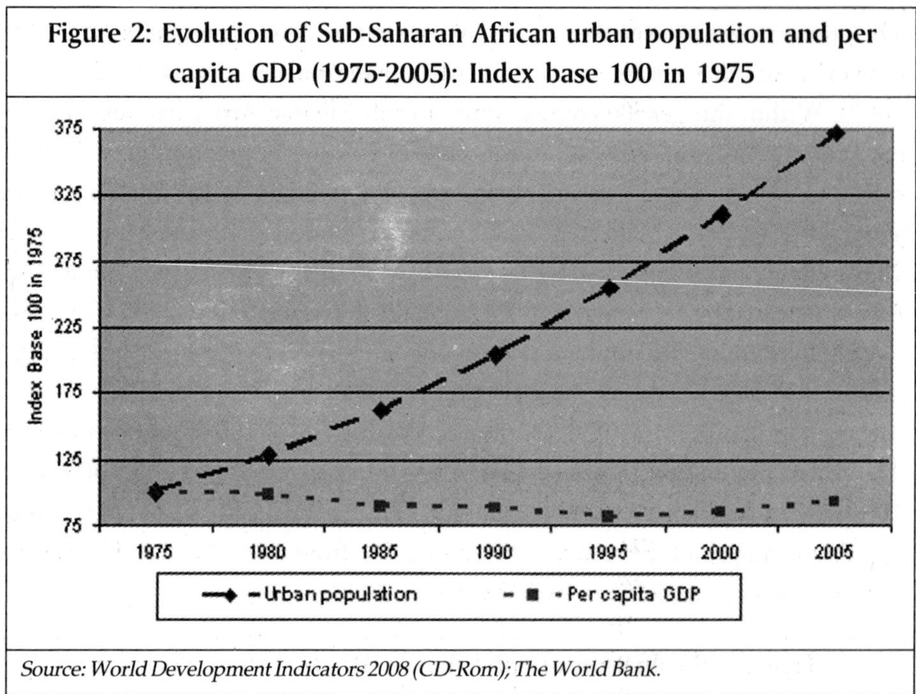

Source: World Development Indicators 2008 (CD-Rom); The World Bank.

The essential feature of current Africa urbanization is that cities have been growing despite poor macroeconomic performance. Consequently, it has been difficult for national and urban authorities to provide affordable housing, quality social services, or sufficient employment to the growing urban populations (Cohen, 2004). Between 1975 and 2005, the region's urban population grew by about 4.5% per year, while at the same time per capita gross domestic product (GDP) dropped by 0.3% per annum (World Bank, 2008), as illustrated in Figure 2. Progressive decay in basic infrastructure such as piped water, electricity, sewerage, and roads have prompted people in large African cities to move to unplanned settlements on the urban periphery (Brockerhoff, 2000; World Bank, 2000). Indeed, one of the distinct faces of urban poverty in sub-Saharan Africa is the proliferation of overcrowded slums and shanty towns characterized by unhygienic environmental conditions (e.g. uncollected garbage, unsafe water, poor drainage and open sewers) which worsen the susceptibility of residents to various health problems (Brockerhoff & Brennan, 1998; Zulu *et al.*, 2002; APHRC, 2002). Recent estimates indicate that about 42 percent of the urban population in most sub-Saharan African countries live in "life and health threatening" homes or neighborhoods where they lack the basic material resources and amenities necessary for a decent standard of living (UNFPA, 1996).

As a result of such unhealthy conditions, rates of child malnutrition, morbidity and mortality are several times higher in slums and peri-urban areas than in more privileged urban neighborhoods, and even than in rural areas (APHRC, 2002; Tim & Lush, 1995). Overall, a recent report observed that urbanization and cities in Africa are not serving as engines of growth and structural transformation, but are part of the cause and major symptom of the economic and social crisis that has enveloped the continent (Cohen, 2004; World Bank, 2000). Even by conservative standards, urban poverty in the region is high and is growing rapidly, suggesting that in the near future most of the poor people in the region will live in urban areas (United Nations, 2007).

The consequences of growing urban poverty on health are now emerging, with evidence of increasing intra-urban health disparities between the poor and the non-poor (Magadi *et al.*, 2003; Fotso, 2006; Tim & Lush, 1995). There are also indications that the rural/urban ill-health and mortality gaps have narrowed in recent years, mainly as a result of stalling and even upturn in urban trends, as a result of urban economic and environmental conditions sharply deteriorating in rapidly growing cities (Fotso, 2007; Gould, 1998). These widening intra-urban and narrowing urban-rural health inequities suggest that the urban bias in the allocation and concentration of health-care resources does not translate into health advantages for all urban dwellers. Despite close proximity to health facilities, urban poor women may not readily use them. Because of lack of stable and regular sources of income, coupled with high cost of living in cities, poor women may not afford to lose hours of economic activities to seek health care services under less than emergency circumstances (Magadi *et al.*, 2003).

Has Sub-Saharan Africa Made Progress Towards Improving Child Health?

Improvements in child survival have been very poor in sub-Saharan Africa. Since the 1990s, declines in child mortality have reversed in some countries in the region; while in others they have either slowed or stalled, making it improbable that the target of reducing child mortality by two thirds by 2015 will be reached. Under-five mortality rate (U5MR) in sub-Saharan Africa varied from 186 (per 1,000 live births) in 1990 to 148 in 2007 (UNDP, 2003; United Nations, 2005; UNICEF, 2008).

This corresponds to an overall decline of about 20% over the 17 year period, or nearly 1.3% on an annual basis, while the MDG targets an average reduction of 4.3% per year. If the region had been on track to meeting the MDG on child mortality, U5MR would be around 88 in 2007. At current trends, mortality rate in children younger than five years will decline by less than 30% by 2015 from the base year 1990, compared to the expected goal of 66.7%.

A recent study on urban sub-Saharan Africa revealed that only five of the 22 studied countries had recorded declines in urban child mortality that are in line with the MDG target; five others have recorded an increase; and the 12 remaining countries witnessed only minimal decline. The authors concluded that failing to appropriately target the growing sub-group of the urban poor and improve their living conditions and health status may result in lack of improvement on national indicators of health (Fotso *et al.*, 2007). More generally, it is estimated that about 90% of the more than 10 million annual deaths of under-five children world wide occur in just 42 countries, 36 of which are in sub-Saharan Africa (Black *et al.*, 2003). Extensive work on child mortality in developing countries indicates that most of these deaths are from preventable causes such as diarrhea, pneumonia, measles, malaria, HIV and AIDS, and the underlying malnutrition (Black *et al.*, 2003; Jones *et al.*, 2003; Bryce *et al.*, 2005).

Figure 3: Current and Projected Trends of Child Mortality in Sub-Saharan

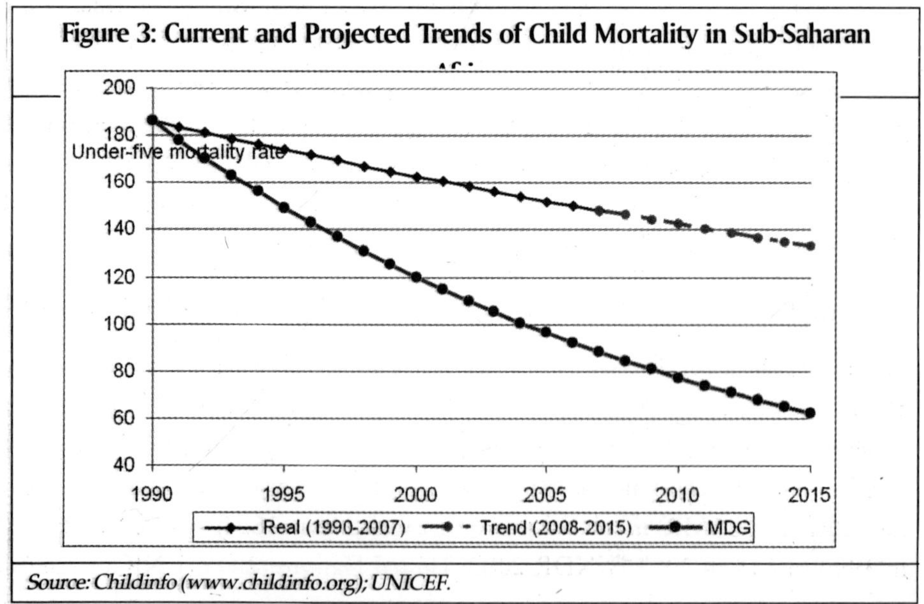

Source: Childinfo (www.childinfo.org); UNICEF.

Indeed malnutrition among children is one of the major public health concerns in developing countries, where it represents both a cause and a manifestation of poverty (UNICEF, 1998; ACC/SCN, 1997; Adair and Guilkey, 1997). The evidence of short and long-term consequences of nutritional deficiencies include increased risk of both morbidity from infectious diseases and mortality, impaired cognitive or delayed mental development, and subsequently, reduced learning abilities in school and poor work capacity in adulthood. There is also growing evidence of heightened susceptibility to poor reproductive outcomes and to obesity and chronic diseases later in life (Gopalan, 2000; De Onis et al., 2000; Adair and Guilkey, 1997; Ricci and Becker, 1996). Ultimately, malnutrition hinders human capital and contributes to the perpetuation of the cyclical nature of poverty (UNICEF, 1998; ACC/SCN, 1997). Conversely, child undernutrition in developing countries is usually a consequence of poverty and its attributes of low family income, large family size, poor education, poor environment and housing, inadequate access to food, to safe water and to health care services (Gopalan, 2000; Peña and Bacallao, 2002).

Unfortunately, progress in child nutritional well-being observed world wide continues to bypass many African countries and population subgroups. Recent data summarized in Table 1 indicate that between 1990 and 2000, whereas the prevalence of malnutrition among preschoolers substantially decreased in Latin America and the Caribbean (-34.0%), Asia (-20.6%) and North Africa (-23.8%), it rose in Eastern Africa (+1.7%), declined only sluggishly in Western Africa (-1.7%) and remains disturbingly high in almost all parts of sub-Saharan Africa (De Onis *et al.*, 2000). As a result, the number of malnourished children increased by 6.7 millions (+18.6%) in sub-Saharan Africa. On the contrary, it went down by 1.1 million (-20%) in Northern Africa; 3.6 million (-34.3%) in Latin America and the Caribbean, and 39.9 million (-23.8%) in Asia.

As rightly stated by Feachem (2000), addressing the problems of inequalities in child health, both between countries and within countries, remains one of the greatest challenges, especially for policies and programs related to the Millennium Developments Goals (MDG). The World Health Organization (WHO) corroborated the focus on improving the health of the most vulnerable and reducing inequalities between population subgroups and stated that "*the objective of good health is twofold: the best attainable average level, and the smallest feasible differences among individuals*" (WHO, 2000).

Table 1: Stunting in Preschool Children in the Developing World (1990-2000)

	1990	1995	2000	Variation 1990-2000 (absolute)	Variation 1990-2000 (%)
			Prevalence (%)		
All Developing Countries	39.8	36.0	32.5	-7.3	-18.3
Africa	37.8	36.5	35.2	-2.6	-6.9
Eastern Africa	47.3	47.7	48.1	0.8	1.7
Western Africa	35.5	35.2	34.9	-0.6	-1.7
Northern Africa	26.5	23.3	20.2	-6.3	-23.8
Asia	43.3	38.8	34.4	-8.9	-20.6
Latin America and Caribbeans	19.1	15.8	12.6	-6.5	-34.0
			Absolute number (in million)		
All Developing Countries	219.7	196.6	181.9	-37.8	-17.2
Africa	41.7	44.5	47.3	5.6	13.5
Sub-Saharan Africa[1]	36.1	39.6	42.9	6.7	18.6
Eastern Africa	17.1	19.3	22.0	4.9	28.6
Western Africa	12.0	13.5	14.7	2.8	22.9
Central & Southern Africa[1]	7.0	6.9	6.1	-0.9	-13.1
Northern Africa	5.6	4.9	4.4	-1.1	-20.0
Asia	167.7	143.5	127.8	-39.9	-23.8
Latin America and Caribbeans	10.4	8.6	6.8	-3.6	-34.3

[1] Not provided by De Onis *et al.* (2000); estimated by the authors.

Source: De Onis et al. (2000).

Against the foregoing backdrop, this paper seeks to revisit the urban advantage in health by examining differences across urban and rural areas in health inequalities. Specifically, its goal is to compare the magnitude of inequities in child malnutrition across urban and rural areas; and compare the intra-urban inequities with urban-rural differences.

2. Data and Methods

We use recent data from the nationally representative Demographic and Health Surveys (DHS) conducted in sub-Saharan Africa in 2003 or later. As of January 2009, 25 countries qualified for the study, including five from the Central Africa;

four from Eastern Africa; seven in Southern Africa; and nine from Western Africa, as can be seen in Table 2. We restrict the samples to the childhood period (12-59 months) and exclude children with missing or inconsistent anthropometric measures.

Table 2: Socioeconomic Characteristics of the selected sub-Saharan African Countries

		Urbanization		Economic		
No	Region, Country, Survey year	% urban population, 2005	Urban growth (1980-2005)	Per capita GDP, 2005[1]	Per capita GDP growth (1980-2005)	Food Production Index -(1980-2005)
	Central Africa					
1	Cameroon, 2004	54.6	5.0	1,993	-0.1	2.6
1	Chad, 2004	25.3	4.4	1,471	2.6	3.1
2	Congo Brazza, 2005	60.2	3.8	3,246	0.5	2.0
3	Congo DRC, 2007	32.1	3.5	267	-4.0	0.4
4	Rwanda, 2005	19.3	8.3	696	-0.4	1.6
	Eastern Africa					
5	Ethiopia, 2005	16.0	4.6	581	0.3	5.2
6	Kenya, 2003	20.7	4.3	1,375	-0.1	3.3
7	Tanzania, 2004	24.2	5.0	933	1.4	2.0
8	Uganda, 2006	12.6	5.5	848	1.9	2.8
	Southern Africa					
9	Lesotho, 2004	18.7	3.1	1,311	2.0	0.7
10	Madagascar, 2003/04	26.8	4.5	834	-1.5	1.6
11	Malawi, 2004	17.2	5.7	648	-0.6	2.4
12	Mozambique, 2003	34.5	6.2	677	1.5	2.6
13	Namibia, 2006/2007	35.1	4.3	4,599	0.2	-0.5
14	Swaziland, 2006	24.1	4.1	4,461	1.4	0.8
15	Zimbabwe, 2005/6	35.9	4.3	1,837	-0.5	1.1
	Western Africa					
16	Benin, 2006	40.1	5.0	1,213	0.4	4.7
17	Burkina Faso, 2003	18.3	6.0	1,061	1.8	4.8
18	Ghana, 2003	47.8	4.5	1,160	0.8	5.0
19	Guinea, 2005	33.0	4.1	1,105	0.7	2.5
20	Liberia, 2007	58.1	4.5	312	-6.8	0.3
21	Mali, 2006	30.5	4.7	1,004	0.5	2.7
22	Niger, 2006	16.8	4.3	602	-1.8	2.5
23	Nigeria, 2003	48.2	5.2	1,520	-0.1	5.0
24	Senegal, 2005	41.6	3.4	1,541	0.4	3.3

[1] GDP per capita, PPP (constant 2005 international $)

Source: World Development Indicators 2008 (CD-Rom); The World Bank.

The selected countries typify rapid urbanization amidst declining economies. In 2005 the proportion of urban population was 17% or lower in Uganda, Ethiopia, Niger and Malawi to 48% or higher in Ghana, Nigeria, Cameroon, and quite surprisingly in Liberia and Democratic Republic of Congo (DRC), with a median value of 30.5% (in Mali). In terms of urban population expansion, annual growth rate reaches 5%-6.2% in eight countries (Cameroon, Benin, Tanzania, Nigeria, Uganda, Malawi, Burkina Faso and Mozambique), and as high as 8.3% in Rwanda. Lower urban growth rates of 3.1%-3.8% were observed in Lesotho, Senegal and the two Congos, while the median urban annual growth rate was 4.5% (in Madagascar, Ghana and Liberia).

Table 2 moreover illustrates the economic diversities of the 25 selected countries with respect to per capita gross domestic product (GDP) and food production. In 2005, the poorest five countries were DRC ($267), Liberia ($312), Ethiopia ($581), Niger ($602) and Malawi ($648). At the other end of the scale, Zimbabwe ($1,837), Cameroon ($1,993), Congo Brazzaville ($3,246), Swaziland ($4,461), and Namibia ($4,599) were the richest top five. The Median value of per capita GDP was $1,105 (Guinea). Economic growth was weaker in Liberia (-6.8%), DRC (-4.0%), Niger (-1.8%), Madagascar (-1.5%), and Malawi (-0.6%), while the top five performers were Mozambique (+1.5%), Burkina Faso (+1.8%), Uganda (+1.9%), Lesotho (+2.0%) and Chad (+2.6%). The median GDP growth rate stood at +0.4% (Senegal, Benin). Finally, the average annual growth in food production varied from 1% or less in Namibia, Liberia, DRC, Lesotho and Swaziland, to about 5% in Benin, Burkina Faso, Nigeria, Ghana and Ethiopia, with a median value of 2.5% (in Guinea and Niger).

Overall, while we acknowledge that these countries are not representative of the entire sub-Saharan Africa, it is important to note that their number, geographical spread (West, Central, East and Southern Africa) and socioeconomic diversities constitute a good yardstick and may allow us to draw some robust inferences.

Child Health Variable of Interest

Among various growth-monitoring indices, there are three commonly-used anthropometric measures that offer a comprehensive profile of malnutrition: stunting, underweight and wasting, measured by the indices height-for-age, weight-for-age and weight-for-height, respectively (UNICEF, 1998). The present study focuses on stunting (or chronic protein-energy malnutrition), which results in young children from recurrent episodes or prolonged periods of nutrition deficiency for calories and/or protein available to the body tissues, or persistent or recurrent ill-health (UNICEF, 1998; Ricci and Becker, 1996). Since height-for-age measure is less sensitive to temporary food shortages, stunting is considered the most reliable indicator of child's nutritional status, especially for the purpose of differentiating socioeconomic conditions within and between countries (Zere and McIntyre, 2003). As recommended by the World Health Organization (WHO), children whose indices fall more than two standard deviations below the median of the NCHS/CDC/WHO reference population are classified as stunted (De Onis *et al.*, 2000).

Defining Household Economic Status

Poverty has been recognized to be multi-faceted, and to exert its influences on health at various levels (individual, household, community and nation). Poverty includes, but is not limited to, inadequate income, shelter and assets for individuals and households, and inadequate provision of infrastructure and basic services such as health services, roads, schools and vocational training (Mitlin, 2003; Peña & Bacallao, 2002). This paper privileges the economic and material dimension of poverty at the household level. DHS data do not provide information on income or expenditures. Thus, along the lines of Gwatkin *et al.* (2000) and Filmer & Pritchett (2001), we use a household wealth index in each country and area (urban, rural). The wealth index is constructed from household's possessions, source of drinking water, type of toilet facilities and flooring material using principal components analysis. The index is recoded as tertiles and the three categories labelled poorest (bottom third), middle (next third), and richest (top third), with poorest as the reference category.

Measuring Inequities[1] in Child Health

Despite the growing number of studies attesting evidence of poorer health among people with less education and income, lower status jobs, and poorer housing (Zere & McIntyre, 2003; Houweling *et al.*, 2003; Kuate-Defo, 1996), there is still debate about the meaning of health inequalities (Braveman *et al.*, 2000; Gakidou & King, 2002; Murray *et al.*, 1999). Kawachi *et al.* arguably state that priority must be given to analysing health inequalities between groups, referred to as health inequities (Kawachi *et al.*, 2002). There is also a great deal of discussion on the appropriate

[1] This paper uses the terms '*inequities*', '*disparities*' or '*socioeconomic inequalities*' interchangeably.

measures to capture such inequities (Wagstaff *et al.*, 1991). The concentration index[2] is increasingly used in the literature on socioeconomic inequalities in health (Houweling *et al.*, 2003; Zere & McIntyre, 2003; Wagstaff *et al.*, 2000). Though this measure takes into account what is going on in all the groups, it is mainly used for descriptive purposes, and adjustment for control variables is not straightforward. The ratios of malnutrition prevalence among the poor and the rich, and the rural and urban residents, are used in this paper as proxies for inequities. The main advantage of this approach is the use of a single number which makes it easier to compare the magnitude of inequalities across populations even though it overlooks the health outcome in the intermediate groups of the economic status variable. This measure is particularly appropriate when a linear trend has previously been observed in the association between the socioeconomic variable and the health outcome under consideration (Kawachi *et al.*, 2002), which is the case of the association between socioeconomic status and child malnutrition in Africa (Fotso, 2007).

3. Results

Sample Description

The selected countries, years of data collection and sample sizes are shown in Table 3. Table 3 also displays the percentage of sample children living in urban areas. The average proportion of urban children stands at 29.4%, with highest values of 35% or higher found in eight countries (Congo Brazzaville, Madagascar, Chad, DRC, Cameroon, Nigeria, Benin and Mozambique); whereas lowest proportions are recorded in eight other countries (Uganda, Burkina Faso, Malawi, Ethiopia, Tanzania, Lesotho, Rwanda and Swaziland (between 11 and 20%). Table 3 also shows about 30% of the sampled children are undernourished. The prevalence of stunting reaches 40% in Malawi, Ethiopia, Chad and Madagascar and even 48% in Niger. At the other extreme, Senegal, Swaziland, Namibia and surprisingly Zimbabwe have the lowest prevalence of malnutrition (between 11% and 20%).

Urban-Rural Disparities in Child Malnutrition

As can be seen in Table 3, the prevalence of stunting is higher in rural areas compared to urban areas in all countries. Urban malnutrition varies from 6-13% in the top five

---

[2] The concentration curve plots the cumulative proportions of the population (beginning with the most disadvantaged) against the cumulative proportion of the health outcome under study. The resulting concentration index which varies from -1 to +1 measures the extent to which a health outcome is unequally distributed across groups (Wagstaff *et al.*, 2000).

Table 3: Child Malnutrition in Sub-Saharan African Countries[1]

		Sample size		Prevalence of malnutrition[2]			
No	Region, Country, Survey year	Total	%Urban	Total	Urban	Rural	Rural-urban ratio
1	Cameroon, 2004	2,449	39.3	25.4	17.3	31.5	1.83
2	Chad, 2004	3,418	44.5	40.2	29.1	42.8	1.47
3	Congo Brazza, 2005	2,977	60.2	21.2	17.9	24.0	1.34
4	Congo DRC, 2007	2,602	40.7	32.1	25.3	36.7	1.45
5	Rwanda, 2005	2,863	19.6	36.3	25.3	38.0	1.50
	Sub-Total Central Africa	**14,309**	**41.2**	**31.4**	**21.7**	**35.9**	**1.66**
6	Ethiopia, 2005	3,155	13.6	40.1	21.0	41.6	1.98
7	Kenya, 2003	3,675	23.5	22.0	17.8	22.8	1.28
8	Tanzania, 2004	5,515	16.8	26.5	17.3	28.6	1.65
9	Uganda, 2006	1,858	10.6	22.0	15.3	22.8	1.49
	Sub-Total Eastern Africa	**14,203**	**17.0**	**27.9**	**17.7**	**29.6**	**1.67**
10	Lesotho, 2004	1,026	17.2	28.8	22.5	29.8	1.32
11	Madagascar, 2003/04	3,488	56.3	40.2	32.9	42.0	1.28
12	Malawi, 2004	6,291	10.8	39.7	28.6	41.4	1.45
13	Mozambique, 2003	6,197	35.1	32.9	20.5	37.8	1.84
14	Namibia, 2006/2007	2,738	34.7	16.6	13.4	18.6	1.39
15	Swaziland, 2006	1,582	20.1	14.2	11.8	14.7	1.24
16	Zimbabwe, 2005/6	3,095	24.0	20.4	16.8	21.6	1.29
	Sub-Total Southern Africa	**24,417**	**28.7**	**31.0**	**21.2**	**33.8**	**1.59**
17	Benin, 2006	9,420	36.6	30.6	24.6	33.9	1.38
18	Burkina Faso, 2003	6,354	17.2	34.0	13.4	37.2	2.78
19	Ghana, 2003	2,459	27.6	21.7	13.0	25.9	2.00
20	Guinea, 2005	1,980	22.1	29.8	15.7	33.9	2.16
21	Liberia, 2007	3,323	34.0	27.6	20.2	30.6	1.51
22	Mali, 2006	8,358	30.2	29.3	17.6	33.8	1.92
23	Niger, 2006	2,878	28.7	47.9	25.2	52.0	2.06
24	Nigeria, 2003	3,264	37.0	34.5	24.5	39.4	1.61
25	Senegal, 2005	2,174	32.6	11.2	6.2	13.8	2.24
	Sub-Total Western Africa	**40,200**	**30.0**	**30.7**	**19.5**	**34.9**	**1.79**
	Grand Total	**93,129**	**29.4**	**30.4**	**20.2**	**33.8**	**1.68**

[1] Among children aged 12-59 months; [2] Based on weighted data

Source: De Onis et al. (2000).

countries (Senegal, Swaziland, Ghana, Burkina Faso and Namibia) to 25-33% in the bottom five countries (DRC, Rwanda, Malawi, Chad and Madagascar), with an average of 20.2% and a median of 17.9% (in Congo Brazzaville). The magnitude of rural malnutrition on the other hand ranges from 14-23% in the top five countries (Senegal, Swaziland, Namibia, Zimbabwe and Uganda) to 41-52% in the five worst performers (Malawi, Ethiopia, Madagascar, Chad and Niger), with a median value of 33.8% (in Mali) and an average of 33.8%.

Urban-rural difference in malnutrition is measured by rural-to-urban ratio. All values are greater than one, indicating that rural malnutrition is higher than urban malnutrition in all countries as stated earlier. The gap between urban and rural areas is lowest in six countries (Swaziland, Madagascar, Kenya, Zimbabwe, Lesotho and Congo Brazzaville). In these countries, rural malnutrition is on average 30% higher than urban malnutrition (ratio of about 1.30). The rural-to-urban ratio reaches between 2.0 and 2.8 in six countries (Ethiopia, Ghana, Niger, Guinea, Senegal and Burkina Faso), indicating large urban-rural inequities in child malnutrition, with rural children more than two times as likely as their urban counterparts to be malnourished. On average, rural malnutrition is on average, 68% higher than urban malnutrition (overall ratio of 1.68).

Intra-urban and Intra-rural Inequities in Child Malnutrition

Of interest to this study is the analysis of intra-urban and intra-rural differences in child health. Table 4 shows the prevalence of malnutrition among the poorest and the richest in urban areas. As can be seen, children from the richest households are consistently better-off than their counterparts from poorest urban households. Whereas the prevalence of malnutrition among the urban poor ranged from 10.2% (in Senegal) to 38.1% (Rwanda), with a median value of 28.4% (Namibia) and an average of 28.5%, malnutrition among the urban rich varied from 3.7% (in Swaziland) to 26.2% (Madagascar), with an average of 12.0% and a median value of 11.7% (Mozambique and Nigeria). As for the urban-rural differences, the magnitude of inequities between the poorest and the richest is captured by the poor-rich ratio. As can be noted in Table 4, the magnitude of intra-urban inequities is lowest (ratio of 1.10 to 1.40) in five countries and highest (ratio between 5.0 and 6.40) in five other countries. In the 25 countries as a whole, children from urban poorest households are about 2.4 times more likely to be undernourished, compared to those from richest urban households.

Table 4: Intra-urban and Intra-rural Inequities in Child Malnutrition

		Intra-urban inequities[1]			Intra-rural inequities[2]		
No	Region, Country, Survey year	Poorest	Richest	Poor-rich ratio	Poorest	Richest	Poor-rich ratio
1	Cameroon, 2004	24.3	6.9	3.52	38.0	22.9	1.66
2	Chad, 2004	36.0	23.0	1.56	49.7	40.6	1.22
3	Congo Brazza, 2005	18.5	16.4	1.13	22.2	23.2	0.96
4	Congo DRC, 2007	33.4	9.6	3.49	33.1	40.0	0.83
5	Rwanda, 2005	38.1	7.7	4.94	44.3	32.5	1.36
	Sub-Total Central Africa	**27.5**	**13.5**	**2.03**	**39.0**	**34.0**	**1.15**
6	Ethiopia, 2005	28.8	5.3	5.40	43.3	39.2	1.10
7	Kenya, 2003	27.6	4.7	5.89	27.4	16.9	1.62
8	Tanzania, 2004	32.4	5.1	6.40	33.3	20.8	1.60
9	Uganda, 2006	23.8	4.9	4.84	25.5	19.5	1.31
	Sub-Total Eastern Africa	**29.6**	**5.0**	**5.98**	**32.6**	**25.7**	**1.27**
10	Lesotho, 2004	27.3	19.3	1.41	38.3	21.8	1.76
11	Madagascar, 2003/04	35.3	26.2	1.35	44.1	34.9	1.26
12	Malawi, 2004	35.3	17.7	1.99	47.2	34.4	1.37
13	Mozambique, 2003	31.4	11.7	2.70	40.1	31.1	1.29
14	Namibia, 2006/2007	28.4	4.8	5.88	22.3	12.4	1.80
15	Swaziland, 2006	18.4	3.7	5.05	19.9	9.8	2.03
16	Zimbabwe, 2005/6	18.6	14.5	1.28	23.5	19.7	1.19
	Sub-Total Southern Africa	**29.6**	**12.7**	**2.32**	**37.2**	**28.3**	**1.32**
17	Benin, 2006	34.9	16.1	2.16	37.9	29.6	1.28
18	Burkina Faso, 2003	21.3	6.4	3.35	40.7	31.5	1.29
19	Ghana, 2003	20.3	5.9	3.43	32.0	19.4	1.65
20	Guinea, 2005	16.5	12.3	1.35	39.4	30.1	1.31
21	Liberia, 2007	29.2	14.1	2.07	34.7	26.2	1.32
22	Mali, 2006	25.0	13.0	1.91	35.1	32.3	1.09
23	Niger, 2006	36.7	12.2	3.00	51.7	53.8	0.96
24	Nigeria, 2003	35.4	11.7	3.03	46.4	26.8	1.73
25	Senegal, 2005	10.2	5.5	1.86	19.6	6.7	2.94
	Sub-Total Western Africa	**28.2**	**12.3**	**2.29**	**37.9**	**30.7**	**1.24**
	Grand Total	**28.5**	**12.0**	**2.37**	**36.9**	**29.8**	**1.24**

[1] Based on the lowest 33.3% (Poor) and highest 33.3% (Rich) wealth index in the urban sample

[2] Based on the lowest 33.3% (Poor) and highest 33.3% (Rich) wealth index in the rural sample.

Table 4 also displays the result of similar analysis for rural areas. In general, rural malnutrition is higher among the poorest than among the richest. Unlike urban malnutrition, there are few exceptions: In DRC, rural poor children seem to be better-off than their rural rich peers (33.1% versus 40.0%); while in Congo Brazzaville and Niger, both groups tend to have comparable levels of malnutrition. Overall, the prevalence of malnutrition among the rural rich varies from 7% (in Senegal) to 53.8% (Niger), with an average of 29.8% in the 25 countries as a whole. Among the rural poor, the figures are 19.6%, 51.7%, and 36.9%, respectively. The poor-rich ratio that measures the magnitude of inequities between the rich and the poor in rural areas is less than one in the DRC, Congo Brazzaville and Niger (as discussed previously); ranges between 1.09 and 1.26 in five countries; and reaches 1.73-2.94 in five other countries. In rural areas of the 25 countries, poorest children are about 24% more likely than their peers from richest households, to experience malnutrition.

Urban-rural, Intra-urban, and Intra-rural Inequities: How do They Compare?

The magnitude of inequities in child health within urban areas, within rural areas and between urban and rural areas is summarized in Figure 4 for the four sub-regions of sub-Saharan Africa. Country-level data are detailed in Appendix 1. Noticeably,

Figure 4: Intra-urban, Intra-rural and Urban-rural Inequities in Child Malnutrition in Sub-Saharan Africa

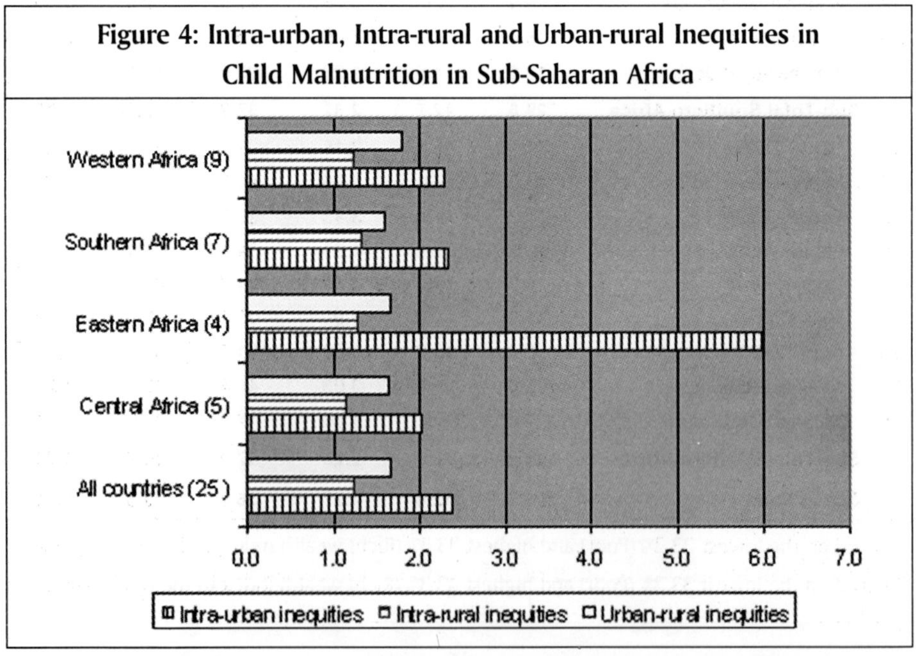

within-urban disparities in child malnutrition are wider that the within-rural disparities and the urban-rural differences in all four sub-regions of sub-Saharan Africa and the 25 countries as a whole.

A striking finding can be noted in Eastern Africa where intra-urban disparities are about 6.0, compared to 1.3 and 1.7 for intra-rural inequities and urban-rural differences, respectively. It appears from the Appendix 1 that this pattern is common to all four countries (Ethiopia, Kenya, Tanzania and Uganda), with malnutrition prevalence of about 5% among the urban rich; 30% among the urban poor; 26% among the rural rich and 33% among the rural poor.

In Central Africa, intra-urban inequities (2.0) though higher than intra-rural differences (1.7), did not differ markedly from the urban-rural disparities; lowest levels of intra-urban gaps in Congo Brazzaville (1.1) and Chad (1.6) offsetting the markedly high levels in Rwanda (4.9) and Cameroon and DRC (3.5). Intra-rural and urban-rural differences did not vary greatly in the five countries. In Southern Africa, three countries (Lesotho, Madagascar and Zimbabwe) display results that seem to depart from the general pattern depicted in Figure 4, with intra-urban, intra-rural and urban-rural differences showing almost similar levels. The general pattern is clearly observed in the remaining four countries where intra-urban disparities reach 5.9 in Namibia; 5.0 in Swaziland; 2.7 in Mozambique and 2.0 in Malawi, whereas the intra-rural and urban-rural inequities are contained in the range of 1.2 to 2.0 (see Appendix 1).

Finally in Western Africa, there are two exceptions to the general pattern. In Senegal, the intra-urban gap (1.9) is lower than the intra-rural gap (2.9) and the urban-rural disparities (2.2). In Guinea, both intra-urban and intra-rural gaps have same levels (1.3) that are lower that the difference between urban and rural areas. In the remaining seven countries intra-urban gaps are higher, followed by urban-rural gaps. Countries with highest intra-urban disparities include Ghana, Burkina Faso, Niger and Nigeria; and higher urban-rural differences are noted in Burkina Faso, Senegal, Guinea, Niger and Ghana.

4. Discussion

This study has examined and documented differences across urban and rural areas in child health inequities, using a sample of 25 sub-Saharan African countries. The first objective of the paper was to compare the scale of inequities in child malnutrition across urban and rural areas. Our results indicate that in all countries and areas (urban or rural), children from poorest households have greater risk of malnutrition compared to their counterparts in the most privileged households. Most studies that have used socioeconomic index (Zere & McIntyre, 2003; Wagstaff *et al.*, 2000) or socioeconomic factors (Madise *et al.*, 1999; Kuate-Defo, 1996; Ricci & Becker, 1996) have reported similar results. More importantly, this study shows that while malnutrition is, on average, higher in rural settings compared to urban areas – a finding reported by other authors (Smith *et al.*, 2003; Fotso, 2007) – disparities between the poor and the rich are, to a large extent, higher in cities than in rural areas. Many studies on socioeconomic inequalities in health have also shown evidence of higher heterogeneity of urban areas compared to rural settings, with the former harboring pockets of severe poverty and deprivation, and exhibiting substantial concentrations of ill-health among the poor (Menon *et al.*, 2000; Haddad *et al.*, 1999; Tim & Lush, 1995; Zere & McIntyre, 2003).

Our results also show that intra-urban inequities in child malnutrition are even larger than urban-rural differentials in malnutrition. This finding is in line with a study conducted by Menon *et al.* (2000), which showed that intra-urban differentials in child stunting were larger than overall urban-rural differences in 8 out of 11 developing countries from sub-Saharan Africa, Asia and Latin America. The fact that within-urban gaps in child health are larger than within-rural gaps, and even larger than overall urban-rural gaps, suggests that using global urban-rural prevalence to characterize child malnutrition may be misleading, since urban average could mask large differentials among socioeconomic groups in urban areas. These conclusions are in accordance with those from a number of studies which have demonstrated the existence of substantial concentrations of ill-health among the urban poor (Menon *et al.*, 2000; Tim & Lush, 1995; Zere & McIntyre, 2003).

Overall, this study suggests that failing to appropriately target the growing sub-group of the urban poor and improve their living conditions and health status, which is an MDG target itself, policies and programs geared at improving children's welfare, including the MDGs, may not meet their national goals. Further, in addition to improving the overall urban and national averages of health indicators, it is important to analyze, track and purposefully reduce health inequities – inequalities that are unjust and unfair, and ethically indefensible (Victora *et al.*, 2003; WHO, 2000), since progress towards the achievement of the health MDGs will not automatically benefit the underprivileged population sub-groups (Wagstaff & Bustreo, 2004). The concern for equity therefore applies even to countries witnessing substantial improvements in child health.

Acknowledgement

The author wishes to thank Ms Rhoune Ochako and Ms Hildah Essendi both from the African Population and Health Research Center (APHRC). The former assisted in data analysis while the latter reviewed the manuscript. The author's time was funded through a Grant from the Welcome Trust (Grant # GR 078 530M).

(Jean-Christophe Fotso, Research Scientist, African Population and Health Research Center (APHRC), Nairobi, Kenya. The author can be reached at jcfotso@aphrc.org).

References

ACC/SCN, 1997. Nutrition and Poverty. Papers from the SCN 24th Session Symposium in Kathmandu, March 1997, ACC/SCN Symposium Report, Nutrition Policy Paper #16, 1997. WHO, Geneva.

Adair, L.S., Guilkey, D.K., 1997. Age-specific determinants of stunting in Filipino children. Journal of Nutrition 127, 314-320.

APHRC (African Population and Health Research Center). *Population and Health Dynamics in Nairobi's Informal Settlements. Nairobi (Kenya).* African Population and Health Research Center. 2002.

Black RE, Morris SS, Bryce J: Where and why are 10 million children dying every year? The Lancet 2003, 361:2226-34.

Braveman P, Krieger N, Lynch J: Health inequalities and social inequalities in health. Bulletin of the World Health Organization 2000, 78:232-234.

Brockerhoff M, Brennan E: The poverty of cities in developing countries. Population and Development Review 1998, 24(1):75-114

Brockerhoff MP. 2000. An Urbanizing World. *Population Bulletin* 55(3).

Bryce J, Black RE, Walker N, Buttha ZA, Lawn JE, Steketee RW. Can the world afford to save the lives of 6 million children each year? The Lancet 2005, 365:2193-2200.

Cohen B. 2004. Urban growth in developing countries: A review of current trends and a caution regarding existing forecast. *World Development* 32(1): 23-51.

De Onis, M., Frongillo, E.A., Blössner, M., 2000. Is malnutrition declining? An analysis of changes in levels of child malnutrition since 1980. Bulletin of the World Health Organization 78(10), 1222-1233.

Feachem RGA: Poverty and inequity: a proper focus for the new century. Bulletin of the World Health Organization 2000, 78(1):1.

Filmer D, Pritchett L: Estimating wealth effects without expenditure data – or tears: An application to educational enrollments in States of India. Demography 2001, 38(1):115-132.

Fotso JC, Ezeh A, Madise N, and Ciera J (2007). Progress towards the child mortality millennium development goal in urban sub-Saharan Africa: The dynamics of urban growth, immunization, and access to clean water. BMC Public Health 2007, 7:218.

Fotso JC. Child health inequities in developing countries: Differences across urban and rural areas. International Journal for Equity in Health 2006, 5:1.

Fotso JC. Urban-rural differentials in child malnutrition: Trends and socioeconomic correlates in sub-Saharan Africa. *Health and Place* 2007, 13:205-223.

Gakidou E, King G: Measuring total health inequality: adding individual variation to group-level differences. International Journal for Equity in Health 2002, 1:3.

Gopalan, S., 2000. Malnutrition: causes, consequences, and solutions. Nutrition 16, 556-58.

Gould WTS 1998. African mortality and the new 'urban penalty. *Health and Place* 4:171-81.

Gwatkin DR, Rustein S, Johnson K, Pande R, Wagstaff A: Socio-economic Differences in Health, Nutrition, and Population. HNP/Poverty Thematic Group, The World Bank, 2000.

Haddad L, Ruel MT, Garrett JL: Are urban poverty and undernutrition growing? Some newly assembled evidence. World Development 1999, 27(11):1891-1904.

Houweling TAJ, Kunst AE, Mackenbach JP: Measuring health inequality among children in developing countries: does the choice of the indicator of economic status matter? International Journal for Equity in Health 2003, 2:8.

Jones G, Steketee RW, Black RE, Buttha ZA, Morris SS, and the Bellagio Child Survival Study group: How many child deaths can we prevent this year? The Lancet 2003, 362:65-71.

Kawachi I, Subramanian SV, Almeida-Filho N: A glossary for health inequalities. Journal of Epidemiology and Community Health 2002, 56(9):647-652.

Kuate-Defo B: Areal and socioeconomic differentials in infant and child mortality in Cameroon. Social Science & Medicine 1996, 42(3):399-420

Madise NJ, Matthews Z, Margetts B: Heterogeneity of child nutritional status between households: A comparison of six sub-Saharan African countries. Population Studies 1999, 53(3):331-43.

Magadi MA, Zulu EM, Brockerhoff M. 2003. The inequality of maternal health care in urban sub-Saharan Africa in the 1990s. Population Studies 57(3): 347-366.

Menon P, Ruel MT, Morris SS: Socio-economic differentials in child stunting are consistently larger in urban than rural areas: Analysis of 10 DHS data sets. Food and Nutrition Bulletin 2000, 21(3):282-299.

Mitlin D: Addressing urban poverty through strengthening assets. Habitat International 2003, 27:393-406.

Murray CJL, Gakidou EE, Frenk J: Health inequalities and social group differences: what should we measure? Bulletin of the World Health Organization 1999, 77(7):537-543.

Peña, M., Bacallao, J., 2002. Malnutrition and poverty. Annual Review of Nutrition 22, 241-253.

Ricci, J.A., Becker, S., 1996. Risk factors for wasting and stunting among children in Metro Cebu, Philippines. American Journal of Clinical Nutrition 63, 966-975.

Smith LC, Ruel MT, Ndiaye A 2003: Why is child malnutrition lower in urban than rural areas? Evidence from 36 developing countries. World Development 33(8):1285-1305.

Tim IM, Lush L: Intra-urban differentials in child health. Health Transition Review 1995, 5:163-190.

UNDP: *Achieving the Millennium Development Goals: Population and Reproductive Health as Critical Determinants.* Population and Development Strategies Series. New York, 2003.

UNICEF, 1998. The State of the World's Children 1998. New York: Oxford University Press, 1998.

UNICEF. Childinfo; *www.childinfo.org*, Accessed in December 2008.

United Nations Population Fund. 1996. The State of the World Population 1996. Changing Places: Population, Development and the Urban Poor. New York: United Nations

United Nations. *The Millennium Development Goals Report 2005*. UN, New York, 2005.

United Nations. *World Urbanization Prospects: The 2007 Revision.* New York: United Nations, Department of Economic and Social Affairs, Population Division. 2004

Victora CG, Wagstaff A, Schellenberg JA, Gwatkin D, Claeson M, Habicht JP: Applying an equity lens to child health and mortality: more of the same is not enough. *The Lancet* 2003, 362:233-41.

Wagstaff A, Bustreo F: Child health: Reaching the poor. *Am J. Pub. Health* 2004, 94:726-736.

Wagstaff A, Paci P, Van Doorslaer E: On the measurement of inequalities in health. Social Science and Medicine 1991, 33(5):545-557.

Wagstaff A, Watanabe N: Socioeconomic inequalities in child malnutrition in the developing world. Policy Research Working Paper # 2434. The World Bank, 2000.

WHO: The World Health Report 2000. Health Systems: Improving Performance. Geneva, WHO, 2000.

World Bank. 2000. World Development Report 1999/2000: Entering the 21st century. New York: Oxford University Press for the Word Bank.

World Bank: World Development Indicators 2008. The World Bank, Washington, DC, 2008.

Zere, E., McIntyre, D., 2003. Inequities in under-five child malnutrition in South Africa. International Journal for Equity in Health 2: 7.

Zulu E, Dodoo FN, Ezeh CA. Sexual risk-taking in the slums of Nairobi, Kenya, 1993-98. *Population Studies* 2002, 56:311-23.

APPENDIX 1

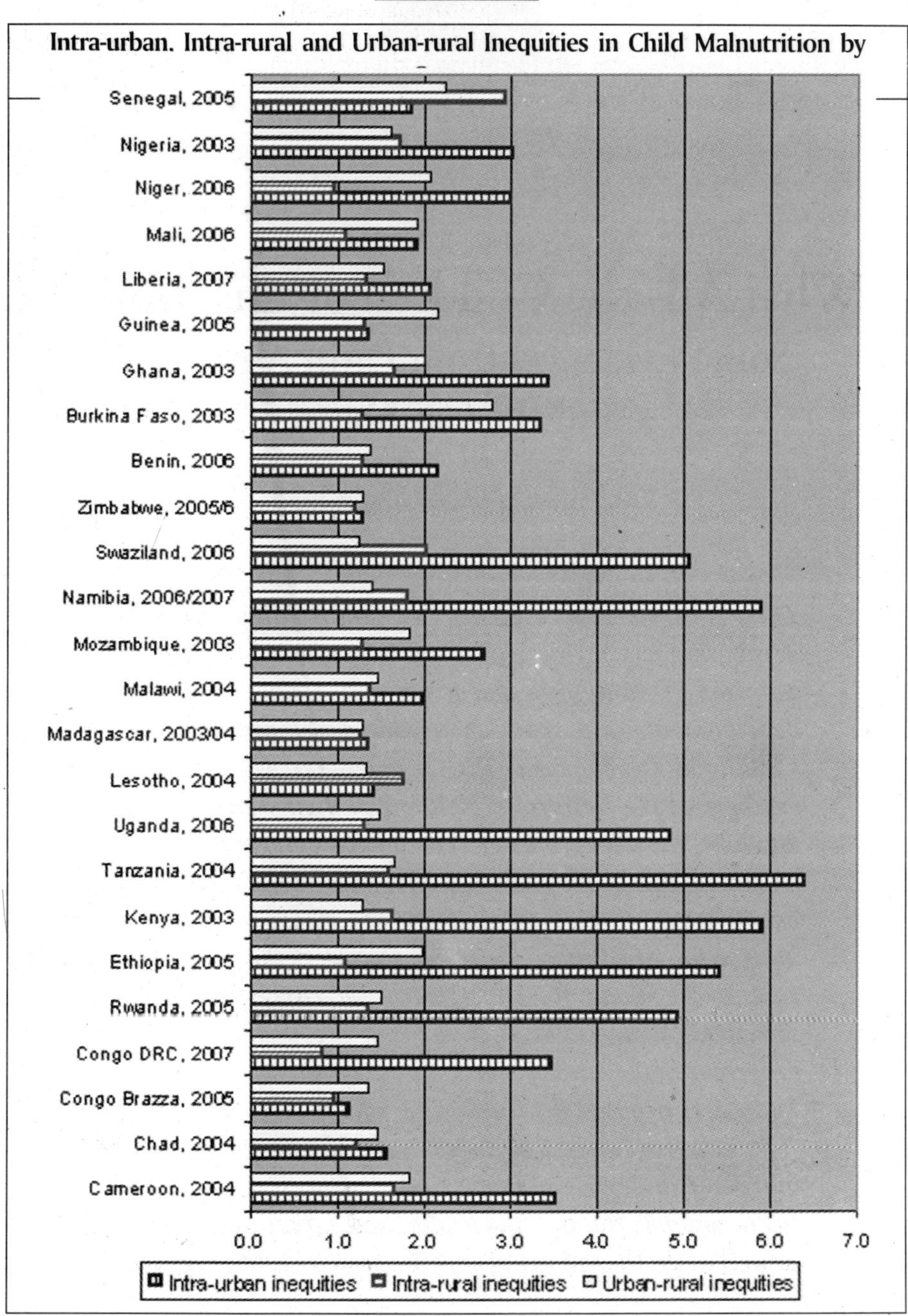
Intra-urban. Intra-rural and Urban-rural Inequities in Child Malnutrition by
Senegal, 2005
Nigeria, 2003
Niger, 2006
Mali, 2006
Liberia, 2007
Guinea, 2005
Ghana, 2003
Burkina Faso, 2003
Benin, 2006
Zimbabwe, 2005/6
Swaziland, 2006
Namibia, 2006/2007
Mozambique, 2003
Malawi, 2004
Madagascar, 2003/04
Lesotho, 2004
Uganda, 2006
Tanzania, 2004
Kenya, 2003
Ethiopia, 2005
Rwanda, 2005
Congo DRC, 2007
Congo Brazza, 2005
Chad, 2004
Cameroon, 2004
0.0
1.0
2.0
3.0
4.0
5.0
6.0
7.0
Intra-urban inequities
Intra-rural inequities
Urban-rural inequities

9

What Ails the Children of this World? Some Evidences from Latin American and the Caribbean

Paramita Mookherjee Nag

There is considerable evidence that young children in many developing countries suffer from profound deficits in nutrition, health, fine and gross motor skills, cognitive development, and socio-emotional development. Early Childhood Development (ECD) outcomes are important markers of the welfare of children in their own right. In addition, the deleterious effects of poor outcomes in early childhood can be long-lasting, affecting school attainment, employment, wages, criminality, and measures of social integration of adults. This paper considers the theoretical case to be made for investments in early childhood, selectively reviews the literature on the impact of ECD programs in the United States, discusses the evidence from Latin America and the Caribbean, and makes suggestions for future research. The focus is on the relation between outcomes in early childhood and measures of household socioeconomic status, child health, and parenting practices, as well as on the impact of specific policies and programs.

The knowledge base on early childhood outcomes is still thin in Latin America and the Caribbean. There are therefore very high returns to comparative descriptive analysis in the region, as well as to careful evaluations of the impact of various programs.

Introduction

Poverty and associated health deficiencies like malnutrition and retarded social cognitive behaviors are a common malady in developing countries, especially among the children. They exhibit all symptoms of nutritional deficiencies and their related health defects. The major problems arise in cognitive development, development in motor skills and the overall socio-economic development. There are some very important markers of child development, namely, Early Childhood Development (ECD). The effect of a negative ECD has a long term detrimental impact and can be manifested as school drop-outs, voluntary unemployment and even anti-social behavior. This article, therefore, focuses on the factors that affect child development in the countries of Latin America and Caribbean where poverty and low development in all spheres, are some of the common factors which are all pervasive.

Investments in Early Childhood

The most important aspect of cognitive ability is the IQ while for non-cognitive abilities it is the faculties of patience, punctuality, self-control etc. Both cognitive and non-cognitive faculties of a person are found to have a profound effect on the schooling of the individuals and the wages received. Some of the factors influencing these aspects are the genetic inheritance, the home environment and also the general milieu. Moreover the stage of development of an individual also has an influence on the perception of cognitive and non-cognitive behaviour. Some abilities are only manifested at a certain stage of life and are also most effective at that point of time. These periods of life are referred to as "sensitive periods". Other abilities only get manifested at certain particular periods, which are often referred to as "critical periods". Skills acquired during sensitive and critical periods are often found to be non-corrective and even if they can be corrected to some extent they might turn out to be extremely costly both in terms of emotions and economics. Moreover, due to the presence of the so called "self-productive" ability of skills and their formations, the skills acquired during one period are found to have a completely separate dimension of their own. For example, self-control acquired during a critical period of a person's life might will make it easier for a person to acquire the skills of tolerance. On the other hand it might make it very difficult to move the person from a perpetual state of self-control to a sensitive state of reaction.

Child development is by far the process through which changes takes place in a child's life and this helps them to understand and analyze the various complexities in later life as their cognizance of ideas take shape. The development of every child is said to start from the prenatal stage and continues through several stages of life (i.e. through the critical and sensitive stages included). It is different from growth in that development takes place through the changes in the complexity and function of life. Moreover, development includes the dimensions of physical growth, of social development of emotional development etc. all these multidimensional aspects are very much woven into the fabric of the development of the child in a proper sequential pattern. The main variance in child development lies in the quality and the sequencing of the cultural events in that particular child's life.

Box 1: Examples of Some Preschool Interventions

The Perry Preschool Program is probably the most-studied preschool intervention in the United States. Between 1962 and 1967, a sample of 128 low-income African-American children ages 3 or 4 who were assessed to be at high risk of school failure were randomly assigned into treatment and control groups. The treatment group received a half-day preschool every weekday plus a weekly home visit—both for eight months of the year, for two years. Project staff collected data on both study groups from ages 3 to 11, and again at ages 14, 15, 19, 27 and 40. Analysis of these data showed that the treatment group outperformed the control group on a variety of measures of educational attainment, including lower grade repetition, higher rates of high school graduation, and higher performance on various intellectual and language tests up to age 7, school achievement tests at ages 9, 10, and 14, and literacy tests at ages 19 and 27. At age 40, those who received the preschool intervention had median earnings that were more than one-third higher than those who did not, were significantly more likely to be employed, had lower fractions of lifetime arrests, and were sentenced to significantly fewer months in prison.

The Carolina Abecederian Project provided a particularly intensive intervention: At birth, children were randomized into a treatment group that received "enriched center-based child care services emphasizing language development for eight hours per day, five days a week, 50 weeks per year, from birth to age five" and a control group (Currie 2001). At school entry, the

Contd...

Contd...

study children were again randomized into two groups, one of which received no further intervention, and another which received a "Home-School Resource Teacher". At age 15, the children who had received the preschool intervention had higher scores on achievement tests, and reductions in the incidence of grade retention and special education. (Children who are placed in a special education "track" are generally more likely to drop out of school in the future.) The effects of the Home-School Resource Teacher were either small or insignificant. At age 21, the children exposed to the Abecederian intervention had higher average test scores, and were twice as likely to be still in school or to have ever attended a four-year college.

Source: ideas.repec.org/p/wbk/wbrwps/3869.html

The above box provides the evidence of the effects of the preschool interventions in the development of the cognitive and non-cognitive ability. Since these early childhood interventions are methodically initialized and motivated by a dedicated and trained workforce with enough funds at their disposal the outcome picture is therefore quite positive.

Child Development in Latin America and Caribbean Islands

Latin America and the Caribbean is very well represented in terms of the literature available especially in the fields of medicine, sociology and economics. Surprisingly, when one tries to look up the health and nutritional status of their children, one finds a sad lack of any documented evidence.

This section tries to bring forth an analysis of enrollment rates especially at the pre-school level.

Latin America and the Caribbean taken as a whole do not appear to be deficient in gross preschool enrollment (GER) rates. The weighted average of the GER is really higher than is expected from a region of their kind of economic status; although this is not significant. But it is found that there is great deal of variations existing between countries. Some of these can be described as "over achievers" like Costa Rica, Bolivia, Ecuador, Guatemala, Jamaica and Peru.on the other hand there are countries like Honduras, Panama, Venezuela and Argentina who can be said to be "under achievers".

Table 1: Enrollment Rates at pre-school Levels

Country	*Gross preprimary enrollment*	*Gross preprimary enrollment: GDP-adjusted (weighted)*	*Gross preprimary enrollment: GDP-adjusted (unweighted)*
Argentina	60.4	-22.6***	-19.6***
Barbados	80.3	-7.7	-2.6
Bolivia	46.3	11.5***	14.9***
Brazil	61.5	7.1	4.5
Chile	77.5	12.3*	10.9**
Colombia	37.0	-6.5	-5.8**
Costa Rica	90.8	30.7***	29.5***
Cuba	108.7		
Dominican Republic	35.1	-11.4**	-11.5***
Ecuador	69.6	32.4***	35.0***
El Salvador	43.9	-0.6	-0.2
Guatemala	51.1	10.2***	11.6***
Honduras	21.3	-12.1***	-9.3***
Jamaica	82.0	29.2**	29.9***
Mexico	75.3	4.9	3.4
Nicaragua	26.8	-5.9**	-1.9
Panama	45.2	-14.3**	-16.2***
Paraguay	28.9	-10.0	-8.2***
Peru	59.5	15.9***	16.3***
Venezuela	51.6	-14.5**	-15.8***
Latin America and Caribbean	**61.1**	**4.3**	**10.9**

Note: Regressions with Huber-White corrected standard errors. * Significant at the 10 percent level, ** at the 5 percent level, *** at the 1 percent level. Sample size is 144 countries.

Source: Wolrd Bank Databases.

Studying the literature available from Mexico, Equador and Brazil a couple of conclusive trends can be noticed. When one tries to compare the performance of the children in Latin America, a large number of developmental deficiencies can be noticed. Moreover poverty and low education of the parents are also found to play a strong role in the defiencies present in children belonging to these socio-economic classes. Another aspect that was discovered was that the effect of a downward pulling economic status became more and more apparent with increasing age of the child.

In spite of recent progress in the Gross Enrollment Rates (GER) percentage of population accessing preschool education, below the age group of six, is seen to vary across sub groups and sub regions and even across countries. In the Latin American countries only 6.5% show enrollment in this age group as opposed to the Caribbean where the GER is as high as 31.5%. Another study reported that around one in every seven children can access preschool education programs.

Policy Directives

According to economic theories it is expected that there would be high returns if investments are made in early childhood. Making up the deficiencies in the cognitive and non-cognitive behaviour later in life incurs a higher cost and is more often than not prohibitive and unsuccessful. In contrast it is found that investing in preschool programs have a higher sense of success and a greater impact among preschool children. In Latin American and the Caribbean, any idea of the relationship between poverty, illiteracy, malnutrition, various socio-economic parameters and child development, the programs and policies are found to be disappointingly lax. Yet there are some opinions, after analyzing the data, that the economic costs incurred due to the lack of cognitive and non-cognitive abilities in the Caribbean and the Latin America is as large as or even larger than that estimated for United States.

Box 2
Careful analytical work is needed to establish the basic facts about ECD outcomes and deficits in the region, and to understand the causal pathways whereby a given characteristic of households, parents, or children determines outcomes in early childhood. A combination of economic theory, experimentation and careful evaluation is needed to identify specific policies and programs that are effective. Recent research from a number of Latin American countries has applied tests of motor skills, cognitive development, and socio-emotional development that have been internationally normed. In theory, norming of the test instruments could have several advantages. Many of the tests have been shown to be correlated with various biological outcomes, as well as with "economic" measures such as school performance and wage outcomes in later life.
Source: ideas.repec.org/p/wbk/wbrwps/3869.html

Evidence from various researches suggests after applying various internationally standardized tests of cognitive development and motor skills in the Latin American and Caribbean countries it was seen that the child development condition is by far much better than the other developing countries of the eastern world. They were also found to have a significant correlation with school enrollment and later on wage differentials.

Some guidelines for policy improvement

- Factor in reducing the gap in child development especially in health and learning and cognitive abilities is attention on micronutrient content of food.
- Preschool food supplements are required to meet the nutrient demand of growing children. Attention should also be paid to pregnant and lactating women whose health determines the development of the baby in later stages.

- Cultural and ethnic characteristics also needs to be taken into account before embarking on a preschool intervention program.
- Incentives in the form of cash and goods are a very good method of luring parents and would be parents to attend programs of intervention like primary health care, vocational training, literacy campaigns etc. Several countries in Latin America and Caribbean have successfully adopted this practice.
- What is also required is increasing public awareness through information programs on food and nutrition, on child care and hygiene.
- The state should invest in education and management of health infrastructure to make it viable and more accessible to the population.
- The people should have access to productive assets that could be used as means of poverty alleviation.
- Agriculture being the subsistence of these regions should be paid more attention. Investments by the government (as subsidies to the farmers for investing) should be made in newer technologies and agricultural inputs like seeds and fertilizers.

Conclusion

In conclusion it must be said that a very careful interpretation is required to understand the intervention results. In the Unites States, the literature shows that, based on the intervention programs there can be large differences in result; Even more so between experimental and non-experimental programs. Therefore such confusing and nearly similar yet different results make it very difficult for the direction of policy intervention. For Latin America and Caribbean, conditional cash transfer programs bear the strongest evidence of carefully designed evaluations. Yet what is mostly lacking is the accumulation and careful documentation of the outcomes of these programs. Therefore, what is eminently required is a huge emphasis on innovative program design followed by careful implementation and a well documented serious evaluation. This should help to build up a strong evidence based knowledge base on Childhood development in the Caribbean and the Latin American Countries, leading to the identification of the correct program to ensure healthy and productive lives of their children.

(Paramita Mookherjee Nag, Faculty Associate, Icfai Research Centre, Kolkata.)

References

Aughinbaugh, A., and M. Gittleman. 2003. "Does Money Matter? A Comparison of the Effect of Income on Child Development in the United States and Great Britain." Journal of Human Resources 38(2): 416-40.

Bassuk, E. L., L.F. Weinreb, R. Dawson, J.N. Perloff, J.C. Buckner. 1997. "Determinants of Behavior in Homeless and Low-Income Housed Preschool Children." Pediatrics 100(1):92-100:

Baum, C. L. 2003. "Does Early Maternal Employment Harm Child Development? An Analysis of The Potential Benefits of Leave Taking." Journal of Labor Economics 21(2): 409-48.

Carneiro, P. and J. Heckman. 2002. "The Evidence on Credit Constraints in Post-Secondary Schooling." The Economic Journal 112(482): 705-34.

Heckman, J. and Y. Rubinstein. 2001. "The Importance of Noncognitive Skills: Lessons from the GED Testing Program." American Economic Review 91(2): 145-49.

Jutte, D.P., A. Burgos, F. Mendoza, C.B. Ford, L.C. Huffman. 2003. "Use of the Pediatric Symptom Checklist in a Low-Income, Mexican American Population." Archives of Pediatrics & Adolescent Medicine 157(12):1169-76.

Powell, C., H. Baker-Henningham, S. Walker, J. Gernay, and S. Grantham-McGregor. 2004. "Feasibility of Integrating Early Stimulation into Primary Care for Undernourished Jamaican Children: Cluster Randomised Controlled Trial." British Medical Journal 29(7457)89: 1-4.

Reynolds, A.J., J.A. Temple. 1998. "Extended Early Childhood Intervention and School Achievement: Age Thirteen Findings from the Chicago Longitudinal Study." Child Development 69(1):231-46.

APPENDIX 1

Child Development Status in India

under ICDS Scheme in India
(As on 31.3.2005 and 31.3.2007)

	2004-05 (As on 31.3.2005)			2005-06 (As on 31.3.2006)			2006-07 (As on 31.3.2007)
States/UTs	Children (6 Months -6 Years)	Pregnant & Lactating Mothers (P&LM)	Total Children (6 Month - 6 Year)& P&LM	Children (6 Months - 6 Years)	Pregnant & Lactating Mothers (P&LM)	Total Children (6 Month - 6 Year)& P&LM	Children (6 Months -6 Years)
Andhra Pradesh	2423099	641395	3064494	2484768	628021	3112789	3255815
Arunachal Pradesh	63183	10776	73959	88494	13629	102123	149241
Assam	1103139	148030	1251169	1260013	148176	1408189	914369
Bihar	2102148	358967	2461115	4019291	835489	4854780	3463544
Chhattisgarh	1416134	363837	1779971	1430228	374103	1804331	1652830
Goa	39731	9279	49010	39571	9267	48838	43726
Gujarat	1643594	277791	1921385	1565728	280575	1846303	1741045
Haryana	933660	236518	1170178	954988	237555	1192543	1119039
Himachal Pradesh	319945	71183	391128	349545	77827	427372	347244
Jammu & Kashmir	182978	39982	222960	273790	69858	343648	424768
Jharkhand	425240	66165	491405	1423868	426069	1849937	1606592
Karnataka	2511867	525114	3036981	2440327	601064	3041391	3075047
Kerala	922125	152937	1075062	902955	162478	1065433	959868
Madhya Pradesh	2841159	668289	3509448	2650862	614455	3265317	3869502
Maharashtra	3304434	518277	3822711	4837317	739851	5577168	5108750
Manipur	0	0	0	178905	38704	217609	259997
Meghalaya	188194	33329	221523	191321	34298	225619	287773
Mizoram	113925	27096	141021	114114	27741	141855	125681
Nagaland	243630	40105	283735	263075	44179	307254	301539
Orissa	3685151	668811	4353962	3717589	661331	4378920	3770595
Punjab	438318	139851	578169	552324	204479	756803	864528
Rajasthan	2711322	609298	3320620	2549408	615434	3164842	2594188
Sikkim	33058	5596	38654	30933	5581	36514	38620
Tamil Nadu	1842967	543264	2386231	1728249	494491	2222740	1862205
Tripura	148205	22088	170293	148205	22088	170293	233427
Uttar Pradesh	6117582	1282818	7400400	7766943	1473434	9240377	16041539
Uttaranchal	372310	85209	457519	378258	90199	468457	538644
West Bengal	3696175	457654	4153829	3880402	463266	4343668	2998314
Andaman & Nicobar Islands	21283	4780	26063	23378	5287	28665	21106
Chandigarh	31723	7624	39347	34563	8418	42981	32958
Delhi	405687	74635	480322	387807	76933	464740	428922
Dadra & Nagar Haveli	12520	2184	14704	11935	2020	13955	11935
Daman & Diu	6977	1898	8875	7094	1792	8886	6694
Lakshadweep	3877	986	4863	4013	965	4978	5758
Pondicherry	31764	9243	41007	29446	9344	38790	29516
India	40337104	8105009	4.8E+07	46717707	9500401	56218108	58185339

Abbr: ICDS : Integrated Child Development Scheme.

Source: *Rajya Sabha Unstarred Question No. 1327, dated on 04.12.2006.& Rajya Sabha Unstarred Question No. 269, dated on 13.08.2007.*

Source: *http://www.indiastat.com/india/ShowData.asp?secid=412017&ptid=17919&level=4*

10

Early Childhood Development and Social Mobility

Barnett, W Steven and Belfield, Clive R

The article examines the effects of preschool education on social mobility in the United States. It notes that under current policy three and four-year-old children from economically and educationally disadvantaged families have higher preschool attendance rates than other children. Increased investment in preschool could raise social mobility Program expansions targeted to disadvantaged children would help them move up the ladder, as would a more universal set of policies from which disadvantaged children gained disproportionately. To them educational effectiveness of early childhood programs would provide for greater gains in social mobility than increasing participation rates alone. The authors observe that if future expansions of preschool programs end up serving all children, not just the poorest, society as a whole would gain. Benefits would exceed costs and there would be more economic growth, but relative gains for disadvantaged children would be smaller than absolute gains because there would be some (smaller) benefits to other children.

Source: From the Future of Children , A Publication of the David and Lucile Packard Foundation, for Volumes 1 No. 2,

Summary

Steven Barnett and Clive Belfield examine the effects of preschool education on social mobility in the United States. They note that under current policy three and four-year-old children from economically and educationally disadvantaged families have higher preschool attendance rates than other children. But current programs fail to enroll even half of poor three and four-year-olds. Hispanics and children of mothers who drop out of school also participate at relatively low rates. The programs also do little to improve learning and development.

The most effective programs, they explain, are intensive interventions such as the model Abecedarian and Perry Preschool programs, which feature highly qualified teachers and small group sizes. State preschool programs with the highest standards rank next, followed by Head Start and the average state program, which produce effects ranging from one-tenth to one-quarter of those of the best programs. Typical child care and family support programs rank last.

Barnett and Belfield point out that preschool programs raise academic skills on average, but do not appear to have notably different effects for different groups of children, and so do not strongly enhance social mobility. In such areas as crime, welfare, and teen parenting, however, preschool seems more able to break links between parental behaviors and child outcomes.

Increased investment in preschool, conclude Barnett and Belfield, could raise social mobility. Program expansions targeted to disadvantaged children would help them move up the ladder, as would a more universal set of policies from which disadvantaged children gained disproportionately. Increasing the educational effectiveness of early childhood programs would provide for greater gains in social mobility than increasing participation rates alone.

The authors observe that if future expansions of preschool programs end up serving all children, not just the poorest, society as a whole would gain. Benefits would exceed costs and there would be more economic growth, but relative gains for disadvantaged children would be smaller than absolute gains because there would be some (smaller) benefits to other children.

Investments in the skills of a nation's citizens can affect both the general level of their productivity and income and disparities in incomes and living standards among them. In this article we examine how current public investments in preschool education for US children are affecting the skills of those children generally, as well as the extent to which those investments are reducing income-related disparities among them—not only during childhood but also when they are adults. We also consider how new investments in those programs might affect children's skills and increase social mobility.

Much research on preschool education and children's skills has been motivated by concerns about income-related disparities in young children's language and cognitive abilities, as well as other measures of their development, including socioemotional skills. Such disparities become evident in children as young as age three and appear to persist—indeed, may even widen—through the school years.[1] Researchers have examined various preschool education programs to learn which might best prevent or reduce these early disparities so that poor children can enter school with skills more nearly equal to those of more highly advantaged children. However, in recent years at least, researchers have paid less attention to an important related question: how preschool education can enhance social mobility by enabling disadvantaged children to achieve as adults' greater socioeconomic success than did their parents.

That poor children begin their lives with lower skills than those of more privileged children is clear. Figures 1 and 2 present estimates of the link between preschool children's skills, both cognitive and social, and the income of their families; they suggest that skills rise evenly with family income. At present federal, state, and local governments in the United States fund a wide variety of early childhood education programs that serve many but not all children. Parents of more advantaged children often pay privately for various preschool programs for their children. Although existing publicly funded programs are demonstrably raising the skills of the children who participate in them, they clearly have not—as Figures 1 and 2 show—broken the link between children's skills and family income. Would increased public investment in preschool education provide additional benefits for children in poverty and help to improve social mobility? If so, what form of investment would be most effective? Some observers argue in favor of limiting increased spending to programs that serve only poor children. Others favor creating a new, universal preschool program that would serve all children alike. A key empirical question related to the latter proposal is whether a quality preschool education program for all children would shift the entire slopes of Figures 1 and 2 upward or would rotate the bottom of the slopes upward while the top remained anchored.

The extent to which preschool policies improve the abilities of all children or reduce disparities in learning and development will depend on the answers to several questions. First, to what extent do such policies alter the distribution of preschool

Figure 1: Abilities of Entering Kindergartners, by Family Income, National Data, Fall 1998 (reported by NIEER from ECLS-K)

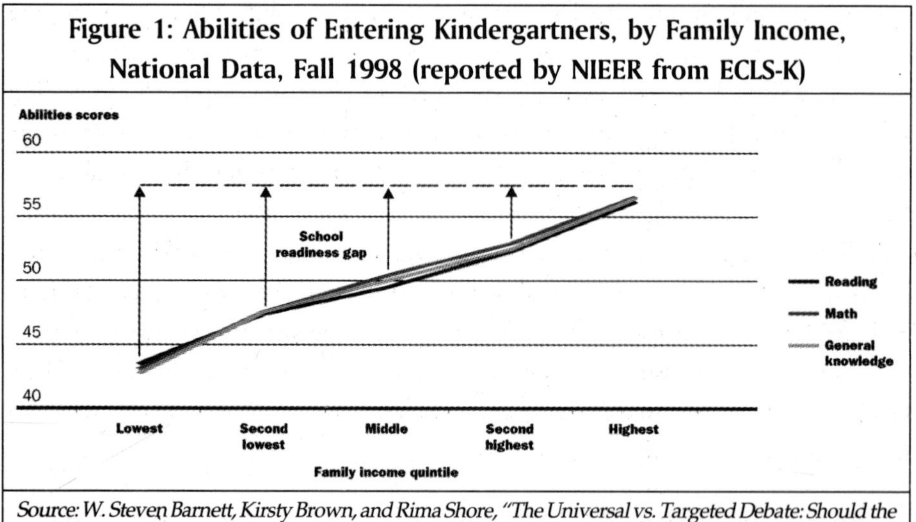

Source: W. Steven Barnett, Kirsty Brown, and Rima Shore, "The Universal vs. Targeted Debate: Should the United States Have Preschool for All? Preschool Policy Matters 6 (New Brunswick, N.J.: NIEER, 2004).

education opportunities? Do they increase the participation of disadvantaged children from low-income and low-education families in effective programs? Do they affect the participation of more advantaged children? Second, to what extent are such programs educationally effective? A subsidiary question is the extent to which preschool programs may improve the abilities of disadvantaged children relative to those of advantaged children. Third, to what extent do these early effects on children's learning and development contribute to their abilities as they grow older, and what aspects of public policy contribute to sustained effects? Is it possible that these early effects may not only be sustained throughout a lifetime but even be passed on to later generations as they affect parents' investments in children?

Figure 2: Social Skills of Entering Kindergartners, by Family Income (NIEER Analysis of ECLS-K)

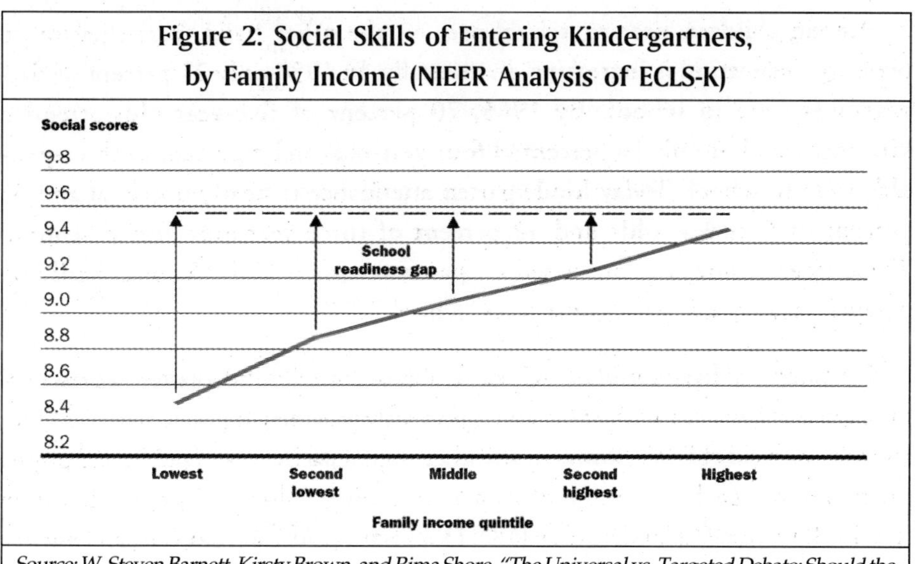

Source: W. Steven Barnett, Kirsty Brown, and Rima Shore, "The Universal vs. Targeted Debate: Should the United States Have Preschool for All? Preschool Policy Matters 6 (New Brunswick, N.J.: NIEER, 2004).

Participation in Early Childhood Programs

Early childhood programs fall into three broad types: early schooling for children from ages three to five, interventions and child care for children from birth to age two, and parenting education. The coverage of the latter two is limited. Before age three, children participate in interventions and center-based care at quite low rates. The largest comprehensive child development program for children under age three (other than early interventions for children with disabilities) is the federal Early Head Start program, which served fewer than 62,000 children in 2003.[2]

Programs for parents also have quite limited participation. A few states—Minnesota, Missouri, and Arkansas—invest in these programs more than others, but even their funding remains limited. Some programs target economically disadvantaged families, others do not. The Parents as Teachers program served more than 325,000 children in 261,000 families in 2003–04, far more than any other parent program.[3] Our analyses of data from the National Household Education Survey (NHES) of 2001 found that just 12 percent of young children had parents who reported participating in a parenting education program or support group (9 percent for parenting education alone).

Among children nearing school age, on the other hand, participation in preschool education is increasing dramatically. In 1950 only 21 percent of five-year-olds were in school. By 1965, 70 percent of five-year-olds attended kindergarten, but only 16 percent of four-year-olds and 5 percent of three-year-olds were in school. Today kindergarten attendance is nearly universal and 65 percent of four-year-olds and 42 percent of three-year-olds attend school.[4] These figures, however, are based on parents' reports and thus necessarily on parents' views about what constitutes "school."

For parents of five-year-olds, "school" is almost entirely kindergarten, a preschool program that has some uniformity and is primarily provided in public schools. Three and four-year-old children, however, attend a complex patchwork of public and private programs that go by a variety of names, including preschool, pre-kindergarten (pre-K), four-year-old kindergarten (4K), Head Start, child care, day care, and nursery school. These programs vary widely in educational intent. Parents of three and four-year-olds typically report private child care provided in classrooms, but not child care in private homes, as school.

Kindergarten

Some children still do not attend kindergarten, which is not compulsory in most states. There is little research on why they do not attend, though the fact that only half-day programs are available in some communities may be a factor for working families. Only in the past twenty years has full-day kindergarten become common, with 63 percent of children who attend kindergarten participating in a regular school day of about six hours. The others attend half-day for two and a half to three hours, frequently in double shifts, some in the morning and some in the afternoon. The distribution of full-day kindergarten is uneven. Of the nine states that require it, all are in the Southeast.[5] Full-day attendance is much more common for African American children (76 percent) than for white (56 percent), Hispanic (60 percent), or Asian children (57 percent).[6] It is also more common among children in poverty (63 percent) than among others (55 percent).[7]

Public Preschool Education

At ages three and four children attend a variety of public preschool programs. For children in poverty, the federal government provides Head Start. State and local education agencies also provide preschool education programs. In addition, federal and state governments subsidize child care, and many children attend private child care centers with and without public subsidies. These programs vary in their goals, resources, standards and regulation, and length of day and year.

Head Start serves about 900,000 children, the vast majority at ages three and four. It serves 12 percent of children at age four, and serves just over half of those children for two years starting at age three. Although Head Start targets children in poverty, self-reported household income data on program participation indicate that by the second half of the school year about half the children served are not poor but "near poor."[8] The reasons why the targeting is less than exact include allowable exceptions to poverty in the eligibility rules, changes in families' economic circumstances after enrollment, and probably some children enrolling who do not meet the eligibility criteria. It also seems likely that some of this apparent difference is due to Head Start's use of family income rather than household income to determine eligibility. Although the overwhelming majority of Head Start children are from lower-income families, it is incorrect and misleading to simply subtract Head Start enrollment from the total number of three and four-year-olds whose household income falls below the poverty line to determine how many poor children are not served. The fact that poverty is a moving target presents a serious challenge for education programs that aim to serve all poor children.[9]

State and local governments support two types of preschool education programs. First, every state serves young children with disabilities in the public schools, though the percentage served varies substantially.[10] States can serve children with developmental delays in these programs, as well as those with identified disabilities. Second, the District of Columbia and forty-one states also fund preschool education for other children (though in a few cases this is only through supplements to Head Start). Most of these programs target children in poverty or otherwise at elevated risk for poor achievement later. Oklahoma and Georgia have for several years sought to provide preschool education to all four-year-olds, and Oklahoma has essentially achieved that goal. Florida moved to join them in 2005, and other states have taken steps in that direction. While state preschool special education programs serve children at ages three and four, most of the states' general preschool education programs focus primarily or entirely on four-year-olds.

These publicly funded preschool education programs are sometimes based in the public schools and sometimes in private programs. In 2004–05 state preschool programs served 6 percent of four-year-olds in special education and 17 percent of four-year-olds, most of them disadvantaged, in general programs, although precise demographic descriptions of the children are not available. The corresponding figures for three-year-olds are 4 percent in special education and 3 percent in other state preschool programs. Additional children attend preschool programs in local public schools using local or federal funds, but no one tracks their numbers nationally.[11]

Child Care and Private Preschool Education

Children also attend preschool programs paid for publicly through federal and state child care funds and privately by parents. State educational standards for these programs are minimal. The only reliable data on the number of children enrolled in all public and private programs are provided by parental reports in national surveys and the decennial census. These data do not allow reliable breakdowns by type of program or funding source, because parents report virtually any classroom as educational regardless of teacher qualifications and educational practices, and many children attend multiple programs or programs that blend funding streams. Publicly funded child care programs generally do not enroll children for an entire school year because enrollment is contingent on family income and parental employment, which fluctuate over time. Thus, while an average of 1.73 million children receive services (57 percent in centers) subsidized by the Child Care Development Fund (CCDF) each month—roughly 225,000 at age three and 225,000 at age four in fiscal year 2004—this does not mean that all of them receive services continuously during the calendar or school year.[12]

At the national level one can roughly estimate the number of children in child care and local public or private preschool programs by subtracting from parent-reported total enrollment the number of children in major public education programs (Head Start, special education, and regular state preschool). At age four, about 66 percent of children attend a center-based program of some sort. The major public education programs account for 34 percent, leaving 32 percent in private programs or locally funded public school programs. At age three, 39 percent attend a center-based program, and subtracting the 14 percent in major public education programs leaves about a quarter of the population (25 percent) in child care and local private or public preschool. Thus, most three and four-year-old children in a classroom are not in one of the major public preschool education programs and most of this residual group is not receiving a direct child care subsidy (13 percent of three and four-year-olds receive a CCDF subsidy, but not all are in centers).[13]

Program Participation by Family Background

Data from the National Household Education Survey can be used to estimate preschool program participation (public and private combined) by various family background characteristics and to explore the determinants of program participation.[14] There are striking differences in participation by income, parental education, ethnicity, and region. From Figure 3, it is apparent that preschool participation declines as income falls until a point just below median income. Thereafter, participation levels off or even rises as income falls. It seems reasonable to infer from this graph that existing public programs are already substantially increasing preschool program participation rates among economically disadvantaged children. NHES data on enrollment at age four in 1991 and 2001 indicate a substantial increase over time for children whose mothers are high school dropouts (36 percent to 49 percent), but these children continue to participate in preschool programs at lower rates than do children of high school graduates (65 percent) and college graduates (70 percent).[15] Clearly there is room for further equalization of access to preschool.

Preschool participation rates also vary by eth-nicity. African American children have the highest rates, with rates for white non-Hispanic children and Asians only slightly lower. Hispanic children have by far the lowest rates. Rates vary by ethnicity partly because the South provides many public programs and the West provides few. Once family background characteristics and regions are taken into account, participation rates for Hispanic children are not significantly lower than for white non-Hispanic children. Rates for African American children remain somewhat higher even after such adjustments.[16]

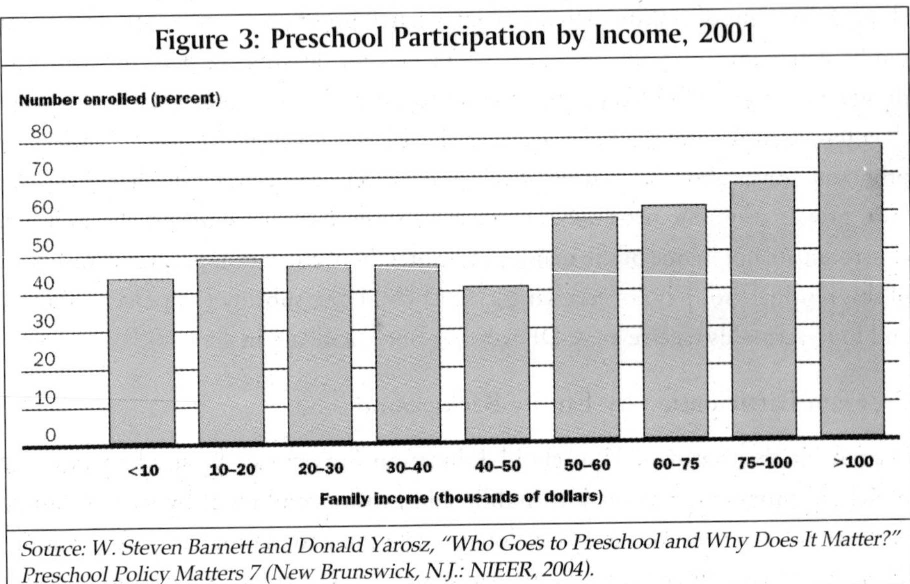

Figure 3: Preschool Participation by Income, 2001

Source: W. Steven Barnett and Donald Yarosz, "Who Goes to Preschool and Why Does It Matter?" Preschool Policy Matters 7 (New Brunswick, N.J.: NIEER, 2004).

Overall, current US public policy increases preschool participation at ages three and four for children from economically and educationally disadvantaged families relative to others, largely through major public education programs. But current programs fail to enroll even half of the children in poverty at ages three and four, or half of the children whose mothers are high school dropouts, even at age four. There is thus tremendous room for public policies to increase enrollment of the most disadvantaged children in preschool education programs. Moreover, the programs that do serve such children—child care and even some public education programs—do little to improve their learning and development. Public policies could also do much more to increase participation rates of children from families up to about the median income. Smaller but still substantial increases in enrollment are possible for all but the wealthiest and best educated.

Influence of Early Childhood Programs on Child Development and Adult Outcomes

How do current programs affect children's eventual educational attainment, earnings, family formation, and propensity to commit crime? And how much more effective might other policies be? Many researchers have examined the effects of various early childhood education programs, with the vast majority focusing on short-term effects on learning and development.

There are literally hundreds of studies of the immediate and short-term effects of child care and early interventions, and their findings have been conveniently summarized in both quantitative meta-analyses and traditional literature reviews.[17] Across these studies, the average initial effect on cognitive abilities is about 0.50 standard deviations, roughly equivalent to 7 or 8 points on an IQ test with a 100-point scale and a standard deviation of 15. Average effects on self-esteem, motivation, and social behavior are also positive, though somewhat smaller. In what follows, we review the best evidence to summarize what is known about how various programs—family support, child care, Head Start, public preschool, and several very intensive educational interventions (which have yet to be implemented on a large scale)—affect children's skills.

Family Support Programs

Although some studies produce larger estimates, the most reliable research—randomized experimental trials—estimates that family support programs improve both cognitive and social development by perhaps 0.10 standard deviations.[18] Randomized trials of many home-visiting programs have failed to find consistent effects on child development, probably because very few of these programs are intensive enough to produce significant cognitive benefits for children.[19] Similarly, randomized trials of comprehensive services delivered in "two-generation" models—so called because they serve both children and parents—have disappointing findings, again because they do not provide substantial direct services to children.[20]

These findings support two conclusions about program effectiveness, both of which are consistent with other reviews of the research.[21] First, influencing child development indirectly through parents appears to be relatively ineffective. Second, a program's effect on child development varies with the frequency and duration of the intervention provided. Even the most intensive family support program devotes far fewer hours to parents than child-directed interventions devote to children. In addition, the costs of such programs, particularly those intensive enough to produce even modest benefits, are substantial, thus likely making them less cost-effective than other preschool programs.[22]

Despite the modest effects of most home-visiting programs on children's cognitive development, one very intensive program has substantially improved the home environment and development of young children. David Olds and colleagues found in a series of randomized trials that a program of home visits by nurses to economically disadvantaged new mothers reduced the number and improved the timing of pregnancies and births after the first child and also reduced the children's need for medical care for injuries and ingestions.[23] Other popular medically oriented programs with similar goals, however, have not been similarly effective in randomized trials.[24] Olds's nurse home-visiting program has also been found to improve modestly both the children's cognitive development (effect size of 0.15 using the population standard deviations for the tests) and parents' report of behavior problems.[25]

Child Care and Early Education

Of all the preschool programs available to directly serve children, only center-based programs in which children attend classrooms or individual tutoring sessions improve cognitive development. The type and quality of activities in these programs vary tremendously. In the best programs children are systematically, regularly, and frequently engaged in a mix of teacher-led and child-initiated activities that enhance the development of language, knowledge of concepts and skills, problem-solving abilities, self-regulation and other socio-emotional skills, attitudes, values, and dispositions. In the worst programs, where little is planned, children wander aimlessly, with few interesting and thought-provoking interactions, activities, or materials, and teachers are unresponsive to their interests or needs. To the surprise of no one, the better programs have the better outcomes.

Studies find that typical center-based child care (as opposed to home or other types of care) improves cognitive abilities by about 0.10–0.33 standard deviations. Most estimates are in the 0.10–0.15 range for cognitive and language development.[26] Evidence is mixed on whether effects are larger when care begins before age three.[27] Some non-experimental studies have found that child care can increase antisocial behavior at school entry, with effect sizes of about 0.08–0.20. The evidence is mixed with respect to whether effects are larger for disadvantaged children than for those from more advantaged homes.[28] Some studies have found that higher program quality, measured in various ways, may lead to small improvements (0.04–0.08) in cognitive and language ability and in behavior.[29] Most child care programs, however, facing minimal government requirements and poor funding, are not designed to improve child development.

By contrast, Head Start, the federal government's largest comprehensive child development intervention, is specifically designed to improve children's cognitive, social, emotional, and physical development, as well as to support their parents in a variety of ways. An excellent recent randomized trial estimates, however, that one year of Head Start has fairly small effects, from less than 0.10 to 0.24 for standardized measures of language and cognitive abilities.[30] This finding echoes that of an Early Head Start randomized trial in which cognitive and language effects were about 0.10 or smaller.[31] Randomized trials of both Head Start and Early Head Start find small decreases (about 0.10) in antisocial behavior. They find no evidence of negative effects on social and emotional development. (The Head Start study did not estimate the effect of Head Start relative to no program, but over and above whatever experiences children received otherwise.)

The best short-term evidence on the effects of preschool programs sponsored by public schools comes from relatively rigorous studies of the Chicago Child-Parent Centers and the universal preschool program in Tulsa, Oklahoma. These studies have found initial effects on standardized tests of cognitive and language abilities ranging from 0.38 to 0.79, depending on the measure. The Chicago Child-Parent Center study found a positive effect on social adjustment in school; the Tulsa study did not look at social development.

The Tulsa study can be directly compared with the Head Start randomized trial on three tests; in each case, the Tulsa effects are several times as large.[32] As with the Head Start study, the Tulsa study estimates effects over and above the experiences that children can get outside the state program, here including Head Start and child care. And the Tulsa study, like the Head Start study, lasted only one year; effects might be larger if the program lasted longer. But clearly, caution is warranted in comparing these two studies.

The Head Start study involves many more children in more diverse circumstances, and the comparison addresses only one program goal (children's cognitive development). It is plausible that the Tulsa and Chicago programs produced larger gains because their teachers were far more highly qualified than Head Start teachers and were also paid much higher salaries. Whereas Head Start requires only that half of its teachers have a two-year degree, Tulsa and Chicago required certified teachers with a four-year-college degree. The Tulsa findings were recently replicated in an evaluation of state-funded preschool programs for four-year-olds in five states, all of which require certified teachers (Oklahoma, New Jersey, South Carolina, Michigan, and West Virginia).[33]

Researchers using data from the Early Childhood Longitudinal Study–Kindergarten Cohort (ECLS-K), a national sample of children entering kindergarten in 1998, have found smaller effects for prekindergarten for disadvantaged children—0.16 to 0.28—perhaps reflecting the poorer performance of state-funded preschool programs overall (many have weaker standards than the Chicago or Tulsa program). The ECLS-K data suggest even smaller effects for child care, where regulations typically require little more than a high school diploma for teachers.[34]

Randomized trials of North Carolina's Abecedarian preschool program and Michigan's Perry Preschool program find that these more intensive interventions involving disadvantaged children up to the age of school entry improve cognitive and language abilities from 0.75 to 1.50 standard deviations—twice the effect of the better state preschool programs and eight times to ten times the effect of Early Head Start and Head Start.[35] These effects suggest a dose-response relationship, in which high teacher quality, small class sizes and high teacher-pupil ratios, and the amount of education given are all implicated.[36]

The Perry Preschool study found positive effects on social behaviors similar to most studies of such effects in the first years of school. In contrast, the Abecedarian study, which examined intensive education through full-day child care over five years, found negative, though transitory, effects on social behavior at school entry. Across studies of early education intervention, intensive research programs, and large-scale public programs, including Head Start, short-term effects average 0.25 to 0.40 for self-esteem, problem behavior, and other social behaviors.[37]

There is relatively little basis for estimating the effects of intensive educational interventions on children from middle-income or highly advantaged families. Few researchers have addressed the topic at all, and even fewer have done so in a rigorous way. The only randomized trial of a preschool program for a highly advantaged population (average IQ was 2 standard deviations above the mean) had a very small sample, limiting its ability to detect effects. Nevertheless it found modest improvements in early academic abilities, at least for boys.[38] The Tulsa study and the later five-state evaluation of preschool education provide some insights, as Oklahoma and West Virginia both serve the general population, not just disadvantaged children, and the other three states also serve populations with some socioeconomic variation. Both studies find that effects are somewhat larger for disadvantaged children.

Long-Term Effects

Though early child care and education have positive initial effects on cognitive abilities, those effects tend to decline over time and in many studies are negligible several years after children leave the programs.[39] The fade-out is most salient for general cognitive abilities, or aptitude, as measured by IQ and similar measures. Only the longest-lasting, most intensive educational interventions (year round, full day over many years), like the Abecedarian program, seem able to produce permanent gains in general cognitive abilities, and these appear considerably smaller than initial gains.[40] Gains on subject-specific cognitive abilities (reading, math, and so forth) seem to be longer lasting, and while these more enduring gains are smaller than the initial gains, they do not appear to fade as often or as much as IQ gains.

Although there is essentially no research on the very long-term effects of typical US child care on educational achievement and attainment, there are many studies of the long-term effects of large-scale public preschool education programs and intensive educational interventions on educational achievement and school progress.[41] Estimated effects on achievement have been highly variable because of differences in research methods and procedures.[42] In the more rigorous studies, which tend to examine the more intensive educational programs, effects on achievement ranged from 0.50 to 0.75 into the high school years. The Chicago Child-Parent Centers study suggests smaller than average long-term achievement gains from large-scale public programs. For Head Start, the initial gains would suggest even smaller long-term achievement gains. Although some studies have found long-term educational gains from Head Start, the effects tend to vary by ethnicity. The lack of such variation in other studies raises questions about these estimates.[43]

Full evidence on long-term effects is reported in Tables 1 and 2. Studies that use cumulative school records data to look at grade repetition, special education placements, and high school graduation provide perhaps the strongest basis for comparing the long-term effects of different programs. They find uniformly positive and statistically significant effects on school progress and placement—effects that have been causally linked to program effects on knowledge and skills.[44]

In an earlier review, Steven Barnett combined data from long-term studies of preschool program effects on grade repetition and special education to compare the effects of intensive interventions, Head Start, and public school programs.[45] Intensive interventions had twice the effect in reducing grade repetition (twenty-four studies) and four times the effect in reducing special education placement (twenty studies) of Head Start and public school programs. Notably, many studies that have looked at these strong indicators of school failure have very similar findings. Given the small size of several of the experimental studies, including Perry Preschool and Abecedarian, the frequent replication of their findings in these other studies strengthens confidence in their results.

Although fewer studies have looked at effects on high school graduation, researchers consistently find positive effects for Head Start, public school programs, and more intensive interventions. It is difficult to feel comfortable with generalizations from so few studies, though grade repetition and special education placement (which have been studied much more often) are strong predictors of dropping out of school. However, the estimated effects of the three intensive programs are quite consistent: a 15 to 20 percentage point increase in high school graduations (not GEDs or other substitutes), from around 50 percent to around 67 percent. The estimated effect on high school graduation in the Chicago study was about 10 percentage points, roughly

Table 1: Effects of Early Childhood Interventions on Education

Change (percent except as indicated)

Intervention and Educational Outcome	Effect
Special education placement	
Abecedarian (ABC)	–48
Perry Preschool	–43
Chicago Child-Parent Centers	–32
Head Start	–28
Public School and Head Starta	–29
Retained in grade	
Abecedarian	–47
Perry Preschool	–13
Chicago Child-Parent Centers	–33
Early Childhood Longitudinal Study-Kindergarten Cohort	Negative effect (reduces)
Public School and Head Startb	–30
High school dropout likelihood	
Abecedarian	–32
Perry Preschool	–25
Chicago Child-Parent Centers	–24
High school completion	
Head Start: white children	20 percentage point increase
Head Start: African American children	No clear effect
College progression	
Abecedarian enrollment in four-year college	3 times as likely
Perry Preschool	No clear effect
Head Start: white children	28 percentage point increase
Head Start: African American children	No clear effect

Sources: Clive Belfield and others, "Cost-Benefit Analysis of the High/Scope Perry Preschool Program Using Age 40 Follow-Up Data," Journal of Human Resources *41 (2006): 162–91; W. Steven Barnett, "Does Head Start Have Lasting Cognitive Effects? The Myth of Fade Out," in* The Head Start Debates, *edited by Edward Zigler and Sally Syfco (Baltimore, Md.: Brookes Publishing Co., 2004); W. Steven Barnett and Leonard Masse, "Comparative Benefit-Cost Analysis of the Abecedarian Program and Its Policy Implications,"* Economics of Education Review *(in press); Arthur Reynolds and others, "Age 21 Cost-Benefit Analysis of the Title I Chicago Child-Parent Centers,"* Educational Evaluation and Policy Analysis *24, no. 4 (2002): 267–303; Eliana Garces, Duncan Thomas, and Janet Currie, "Longer-Term Effects of Head Start,"* American Economic Review *92 (2002): 999–1012; Janet Currie, "Early Childhood Programs,"* Journal of Economic Perspectives *15 (2001): 213–38; Centers for Disease Control and Prevention, "Community Interventions to Promote Healthy Social Environments. Early Childhood Development and Family Housing,"* Morbidity and Mortality Weekly Report *51 (2002); Judy Temple, Arthur Reynolds, and Wendy Miedel, "Can Early Intervention Prevent High School Drop-Out? Evidence from the Chicago Child-Parent Centers,"* Urban Education *35 (2000): 31–56.*

a. Nine-study average. b. Ten-study average.

half that of the Perry Preschool and Abecedarian programs. A few studies have focused on Head Start, with inconsistent results: one finds high school graduation rates increased for girls by 15 percentage points, another finds a 20 percentage point increase for whites only. Such gains seem improbable, given the very small initial effects found in the national impact study.

The Abecedarian study, but not the Perry Preschool study, found gains in college enrollment. It is difficult to know how to interpret this finding. The Perry Preschool sample was much more educationally disadvantaged than the Abecedarian sample. It may have been that college was just too far beyond their reach, given their starting abilities, whereas the Abecedarian children were close enough that the boost they received made college possible for a significant share.

Although relatively few in number, most studies that assessed long-term effects on social behavior found positive (though not always statistically significant) effects, and no study reported increased aggression beyond first grade.[46] Five studies of educational interventions that investigated long-term effects on social behavior found beneficial effects on classroom behavior, social adjustment, and crime.[47] These include two of the three studies that linked elevated aggression with full-time child care that began in infancy.[48] The third, the Abecedarian study, found no long-term effect on crime and delinquency, though rates were relatively low for both groups.[49] The strongest effects on crime were found in the Perry Preschool study, where baseline rates for the control group were quite high: the number of arrests was cut by 50 percent. In the Chicago study, the number of arrests by age eighteen was cut by 40 percent, while the share of people ever arrested was cut by a third (or 8 percentage points), from 25 percent to 17 percent. Data on Head Start are limited to two studies: one finds a 12 percentage point reduction crime for African Americans only; the other, a 10 percentage point reduction for girls only.[50]

There is little research on the effects of preschool programs on later fertility behavior.

The model programs show strong effects, and family support interventions have reported direct effects on fertility behavior of the mothers. Effects are reported in Table 2.

Table 2: Effects of Early Childhood Interventions on Adolescent and Adult Behaviors

Percent except as indicated

Intervention and behaviors	Control or comparison group	Group receiving early childhood program
Teenage parenting rates		
Abecedarian	45	26
Perry Preschool	37	26
Chicago Child-Parent Centers	27	20
Well-being		
Health problem (Perry Preschool)	29	20
Drug user (Abecedarian)	39	18
Needed treatment for addiction (Perry Preschool)	34	22
Abortion (Perry Preschool)	38	16
Abuse/neglect by age 17 (Chicago Child-Parent Centers)	9	6
Criminal activity		
Number of felony violent assaults (Perry Preschool)	0.37	0.17
Juvenile court petitions (Chicago Child-Parent Centers)	25	16
Booked or charged with a crime (Head Start)		12 percentage points lower
Net earnings gain from participating in early childhood programs		
Abecedarian	$35,531	
Perry Preschool Program	$38,892	
Chicago Child-Parent Centers	$30,638	
Head Start	No effect	

Sources: Belfield and others (see Table 1); Masse and Barnett (see table 1); Arthur Reynolds and others (see Table 1); Garces and others (see Table 1); Currie (see Table 1); Centers for Disease Control and Prevention (see Table 1).

Finally, direct effects have been found on employment and earnings. One study found that Head Start raised earnings, but only for white children whose parents were high school dropouts. The model program effects, shown in Table 2, may be considered upper bounds on the earnings gain from state-funded preschool.

Program Design and Effectiveness

From the evidence reviewed so far, it should be clear that some preschool programs are more effective than others. A rough ranking from least to most educationally effective under current policies is typical child care and family support programs, Head Start and many state preschool programs, state preschool programs with high standards (far from all of them), and intensive educational interventions. On average, state preschool programs differ little from Head Start in their effects on child development, but states with lower standards likely have worse outcomes and those with higher standards, better outcomes. A reasonable conclusion is that auspices *per se* have little to do with program effectiveness, once goals, standards, and resources are taken into account. The pattern is clearest for short-term outcomes, where the most data are available. It is less clear for long-term effects on educational attainment and adult social and economic outcomes, where fewer data are available. It does not seem plausible that programs with very weak initial effects would have proportionately larger effects on adult outcomes than on short and medium-term outcomes.

Given the limits of the data, it appears best to produce a range of estimates of the programs' effects on cognitive and social-emotional development. An upper bound would be effects of the size produced by the Perry Preschool and Abecedarian programs. One then might expect high-quality interventions in public preschool programs to produce effects of half that size. Less educationally intensive public programs, including Head Start *under current policies,* would be likely to produce effects of one-quarter or less, and possibly only one-tenth, of those of Perry and Abecedarian. Regarding effects on children who are not disadvantaged, based on the meager evidence we consider two different scenarios. One is that effects are half those estimated for disadvantaged children. The other is that effects on the educational attainment of advantaged children are essentially zero. Given the small effects of child care, if programs effectively target disadvantaged children, then effects on other children are irrelevant.

In designing policy proposals to improve preschool programs, it should be kept in mind that the most effective educational interventions were more intensive in two senses. First, they had highly qualified, well-paid teachers and high ratios of teachers to children. Second, some provided a large number of hours of intervention over two to nearly five years. The Perry program provided one teacher (not an assistant) for every six or seven students. Although it operated only half-day during the school year (and most, but not all, children attended for two years), teachers visited each child at home weekly. The Abecedarian program had a teacher and an aide for every twelve children and operated for up to ten hours a day, fifty weeks a year, over almost five years. This pattern can hardly be considered surprising and is consistent with other evidence. It posits that more highly educated, better prepared, better supervised, and better compensated teachers are more effective.[51] Smaller class sizes and better teacher-student ratios result in better teaching and more individual attention, which produce larger gains in achievement and school success.[52] Finally, more hours of effective interventions produce larger effects.

The Effects of Early Childhood Education on Social Mobility

The above evidence on access and outcomes suggests the following conclusions about the extent to which preschool, as it now stands, affects social mobility by breaking down the links between parental socioeconomic status and behaviors and children's status and behaviors.

Although current public programs move in the direction of equalizing preschool opportunities across races and income levels, they fall considerably short of their goal. Preschool opportunities are not close to equal for Hispanic children. Nor are preschool opportunities equal when mother's education is considered, or when the quality of the different programs is accounted for, or when children aged three as well as four are included. Furthermore, Head Start funding is so limited that it precludes serving most of the eligible population, and public preschool program coverage varies greatly from state to state. Thus many opportunities exist for expanding preschool, but the form of that expansion is critical, as we discuss below.

In addition, broader questions might be raised about the extent to which current preschool programs integrate social groups. Given the separation of children in Head Start and other compensatory programs, preschool programs do not appear to be structured so as to allow disadvantaged children to benefit from long-term exposure to other children. And where preschool programs are tied to local public schools, residential patterns may also limit socioeconomic integration.

assault.[63] The effects appear to be significant, if only because any reduction in criminal activity conveys substantial economic benefits.

Other second-generation effects are probably weaker. There may be some effect on second-generation earnings, to the extent that preschool weakens the link between parents' and children's incomes.[64] Finally, preschool may affect educational attainment across generations. Both mother's and father's education are statistically significant influences on a child's graduation and years of schooling.[65] One extra year of parental schooling is associated, on average, with 0.29 years of offspring attainment.[66]

Although these arguments are plausible, there is no direct evidence on the benefits to subsequent generations from either state or model preschool programs. (Because the sample sizes in the model programs are so small, it is typically not possible to identify second-generation effects.)[67] Moreover, because such benefits would be a long time in the future, they would need to be discounted (valued less relative to immediate benefits). Applying a social discount rate of 3.5 percent, we find that any monetary gain for a child is worth half that of a gain in the same domain to the actual participant. So, even with perfect heritability, the effects on social mobility are half as strong for the second generation.

In summary, there is some evidence that direct and indirect heritability effects are significant, though there is insufficient research from which to generalize to an anticipated effect of participation in early childhood education programs. A recent simulation model, however, suggests that these effects are meaningful.

Diego Restuccia and Carlos Urrutia generate a four-period model of parent-child investments to determine social mobility across generations, contingent on increased public spending on elementary and secondary education, and separately, on higher education.[68] In their policy simulations, they find that increased spending on elementary and secondary education (which can include prekindergarten and kindergarten) raises social mobility. The logic is relatively straightforward. Increased public spending on the early years of schooling—in the model, the increased spending is used for a universal program of preschooling for all children, regardless of family background—eases the burden of borrowing for educational investments for poorer families (although it also motivates some wealthier parents to switch from private to public schools). The children of poorer families will then go on to college, and although they will drop out at relatively high rates, the children who finish will increase the number of college graduates from low-income backgrounds. In the model, intergenerational earnings and education correlations both fall as a result. Assuming an increase in public spending on early education of $90 billion—sufficient to fund preschool for all children for approximately two years—earnings correlations across generations should fall from 0.40 to 0.36 (a perfect correlation would be 1, no correlation at all would be 0) and education correlations across generations should fall from 0.35 to 0.28.

Relative to other educational investments in the model, these effects are substantial. Spending on higher education in the model, for example, has zero or even a negative effect on these earnings correlations: subsidies awarded to a college student do not greatly affect the student's ability to graduate from college.[69] However, in this model the spending on early education would do little to raise educational attainment (college enrollment and completion) for the lowest income quintile. Its main effect would be to equalize college enrollment rates for the three middle quintiles of family income.

Targeted or Universal Preschooling?

The above discussion assumes a trend toward universal preschooling, or at least that any program expansion would be distributed in the same way as the present system. In part, that assumption reflects widespread political support for universal programs and the practical challenges of more accurately targeting programs to the disadvantaged. A universal program should still reduce inequalities, because it benefits low-income and minority children more than it does advantaged children, but the effects (especially at current quality levels) on relative socioeconomic position may not be strong.

In theory, programs targeted at the most disadvantaged children would increase social mobility the most. A targeted program would obviously generate benefits for those who enrolled. Indeed, existing public preschool programs do raise social mobility. But many children who would enroll in a new targeted program would either be white non-Hispanic or Hispanic or be in the lower-middle quartile of income distribution. Thus Hispanic children might gain more than African American children (who have much higher preschool participation rates), and children in poverty would not benefit much more than children in families with higher but still modest incomes. Moreover, it may not be easy to identify the enrollees who might benefit most from a targeted program (particularly children of mothers who are high school dropouts) and exhort them to participate.[70] Screening, regulating, and monitoring eligibility would also raise unit costs. With imperfect targeting, many disadvantaged children would miss out on programs. If the challenges of targeting could be overcome, however, social mobility effects might be greater.

Because many low-income and minority children are already enrolled in Head Start and other programs, another way to raise social mobility would be to upgrade the existing program. Janet Currie and Matthew Nei-dell have found that increased spending on Head Start does appear to enhance outcomes.[71] Also, state programs (most of which are funded at rates below Head Start) might be upgraded. Here the challenge is to get sufficient resources for high-quality targeted programs. Another option is to expand Head Start and state programs to serve all children for two years, which would generate stronger effects. At present most children attend such programs for only one year.

The dilemma is the old efficiency-equity trade-off. A targeted program would have a greater impact on social mobility, but it would not generate as high a public return on investment as a universal program.[72] If a program targeted to the lowest quintile is only 50 percent accurate—that is, if half of the participants are not from the lowest quintile—then it would generate smaller returns than a universal program (even as the average benefits from such a program would be significantly lower). Universal programs are also much more likely to garner political support, as well as generate spillover benefits such as better school discipline. And any fiscal savings these programs yield will be passed on to taxpayers. Thus a useful strategy for increasing social mobility might be to target within a universal system by providing more intensive programs, with smaller classes and longer hours, to disadvantaged children. However, the amount of extra resources needed to yield sufficient social mobility cannot be easily specified.

Conclusions

US preschool programs are effective across a wide set of outcomes. But participation rates are lower for children with lower incomes and low parental education, for

Hispanics, and for those residing in the western states than for other children. Together, these facts suggest that increased investment in preschool could raise social mobility. Program expansions targeted to disadvantaged children would help them move up the ladder, as would a more universal set of policies from which disadvantaged children gained disproportionately. Increasing the educational effectiveness of these programs would provide for greater gains in social mobility than would increasing participation rates alone. At the same time, expectations of what can be accomplished on this front should be modest.

Under current policies, preschool participation rates are not vastly different across races and income levels. Future expansions may end up serving all children, not just the poorest. In this scenario, society as a whole would gain. Benefits would exceed costs, and there would be more economic growth and thus more upward mobility, but not necessarily substantially greater opportunities for those at the bottom of the economic ladder.

(W Steven Barnett is director of the National Institute for Early Education Research, Rutgers University.

Clive R Belfield is assistant professor in the Department of Economics, Queens College, City University of New York.)

Endnotes

1 See Jack Shonkoff and Deborah Phillips, *From Neurons to Neighborhoods: The Science of Early Childhood Development* (Washington: National Academy Press, 2000); Donald Rock and A. Jackson Stenner, "Assessment Issues in the Testing of Children at School Entry," *Future of Children* 15, no. 1 (2005): 15–34.

2 Administration for Children and Families, "Head Start Program Fact Sheet: Fiscal Year 2006" (2006), *www.acf.hhs.gov/programs/hsb/research/2006.htm* (accessed April 13, 2006).

3 Parents as Teachers, "2003–04 Parents as Teachers Born to Learn Annual Program Report Summary" (2004), *www.parentsasteachers.org/atf/cf/%7B00812ECA-A71B-4C2C-8FF3-8F16A5742EEA%7D/PAT%20NEWS%20FINAL%20VERSION%20-%20National%20Annual%20Program%20Report%20Summary.pdf* (accessed April 13, 2006).

4 W. Steven Barnett and Donald J. Yarosz, "Who Goes to Preschool and Why Does It Matter?" *Preschool Policy Matters* 7 (New Brunswick, N.J.: National Institute for Early Education Research, 2004).

5 Debra J. Ackerman, W. Steven Barnett, and Kenneth Robin, "Making the Most of Kindergarten: Present Trends and Future Issues in the Provision of Full-Day Programs," *NIEER Policy Report* (March 2005), *http://nieer.org/docs/index.php?DocID=118* (accessed April 13, 2006).

6 John Wirt and others, *The Condition of Education 2004: 111* (U.S. Department of Education, 2004).

7 Jill Walston and Jerry West, *Full-Day and Half-Day Kindergarten in the United States: Findings from the Early Childhood Longitudinal Study, Kindergarten Class of 1998–99* (Washington: National Center for Education Statistics, 2004), p. 73. There are some surprising differences between this study and the Current Population Survey in estimates of full-day kindergarten attendance by ethnicity and other background characteristics of the children.

8 We analyzed data from the 2001 National Household Education Survey for reported Head Start attendance by income. Although there appears to be substantial error in reported Head Start participation, those whose participation can be verified do not significantly differ in income from those whose participation cannot be verified. Mary Hagedorn and others, *National Household Education Surveys Program of 2001: Data Files and Electronic Codebook,* NCES 2003078 (U.S. Department of Education, 2003).

9 W. Steven Barnett, Kirsty Brown, and Rima Shore, "The Universal vs. Targeted Debate: Should the United States Have Preschool for All?" *Preschool Policy Matters* 6 (New Brunswick, N.J.: National Institute for Early Education Research, 2003).

10 W. Steven Barnett and others, *The State of Preschool: 2005 State Preschool Yearbook* (New Brunswick, N.J.: NIEER, 2006).

11 Ibid.

12 Administration for Children and Families, "FFY 2004 CCDF Data Tables and Charts (Preliminary Estimates)" (2005), *www.acf.hhs.gov/programs/ccb/research/04acf800/list.htm* (accessed April 13, 2006).

13 Barnett and Yarosz, "Who Goes to Preschool?" (see note 4); Barnett and others, *The State of Preschool* (see note 10).

14 Hagedorn and others, *National Household Education Surveys Program of 2001* (see note 8).

15 Barnett and Yarosz, "Who Goes to Preschool?" (see note 4).

16 Ibid.

17 Ruth McKey and others, *The Impact of Head Start on Children, Families, and Communities* (Washington: Head Start Evaluation Synthesis and Utilization Project, 1985);

Craig Ramey, Donna Bryant, and Tanya Suarez, "Preschool Compensatory Education and the Modifiability of Intelligence: A Critical Review," in *Current Topics in Human Intelligence*, edited by Douglas Detterman (Norwood, N.J.: Ablex, 1985), pp. 247–96; Michael Guralnick and Forrest C. Bennett, *The Effectiveness of Early Intervention for At-Risk and Handicapped Children* (New York: Academy Press, 1987); Michael Guralnick, "Second Generation Research on the Effectiveness of Early Intervention," *Early Education and Development* 4, no. 4 (1993): 366–78; Jack Shonkoff and Samuel Meisels, *Handbook of Early Childhood Intervention* (Cambridge University Press, 2000).

18 Deanna Gomby, Patti Culross, and Richard Behrman, "Home Visiting: Recent Program Evaluations—Analysis and Recommendations," *Future of Children* 9, no.1 (1999): 4–26.

19 Amy Baker, Chaya Piotrkowski, and Jeanne Brooks-Gunn, "The Home Instruction Program for Preschool Youngsters (HIPPY)," *Future of Children* 9, no. 1 (1999): 116–33; Gloria Boutte, "The Effects of Home Intervention on Rural Children's Home Environments, Academic Self-Esteem, and Achievement Scores" (Ann Arbor, Mich.: UMI Dissertation Services, 1992); Mary Wagner and Serena Clayton, "The Parents as Teachers Program: Results from Two Demonstrations," *Future of Children* 9, no. 1 (1999): 91–116; Sandra Scarr and Kathleen McCartney, "Far from Home: An Experimental Evaluation of the Mother-Child Home Program in Bermuda," *Child Development* 59 (1988): 531–43; Christine Powell and Sandra Grantham-McGregor, "Home Visiting of Varying Frequency and Child Development," *Pediatrics* 84 (1989): 157–64.

20 Robert St. Pierre and Jean Layzer, "Using Home Visits for Multiple Purposes: The Comprehensive Child Development Program," *Future of Children* 9, no.1 (1989): 134–51.

21 Glenn Casto and Anne Lewis, "Parent Involvement in Infant and Preschool Programs," *Journal of the Division of Early Childhood* 9 (1984): 49–56; Donna Bryant and Craig Ramey, "Prevention-Oriented Infant Education Programs," *Journal of Children in Contemporary Society* 7 (1987): 17–35.

22 Robert St. Pierre, Jean Layzer, and Helen Barnes, "Regenerating Two-Generation Programs," in *Early Care and Education for Children in Poverty: Promises, Programs, and Long-Term Results*, edited by W. Steven Barnett and Sarane Boocock (SUNY Press, 1998), pp. 99-121.

23 David Olds and others, "Prenatal and Infancy Home Visitation by Nurses: Recent Findings," *Future of Children* 9, no.1 (1999): 44–66.

24 Deanna Gomby, *Home Visitation in 2005: Outcomes for Children and Parents* (Washington: Committee for Economic Development, 2005), *www.ced.org/projects/kids.shtml* (accessed February 12, 2006).

25 David Olds and others, "Effects of Nurse Home-Visiting on Maternal Life Course and Child Development: Age 6 Follow-Up Results of a Randomized Trial," *Pediatrics* 114 (2004): 1550–59.

26 Sandra Scarr, Marlene Eisenberg, and Kirby Deater-Deckard, "Measurements of Quality in Child Care Centers," *Early Childhood Research Quarterly* 9, no 2 (1994): 131–52; Sandra Hofferth, "Child Care in the First Three Years of Life and Preschoolers' Language and Behavior," paper presented at the biennial meeting of the Society for Research in Child Development, Albuquerque, N.M., April 1989; Katherine Magnuson, Chris Ruhm, and Jane Waldfogel, "Does Prekindergarten Improve School Preparation and Performance?" *Economics of Education Review* (2006, forthcoming); NICHD Early Child Care Research Network and Greg Duncan, "Modeling the Impacts of Child Care Quality on Children's Preschool Cognitive Development," *Child Development* 74, no. 5 (2003): 1454–75.

27 Bengt-Erik Andersson, "Effects of Public Day Care—A Longitudinal Study," *Child Development* 60 (1989): 857–66; Tiffany Field, "Quality Infant Day Care and Grade School Behavior and Performance," *Child Development* 62 (1991): 863–70.

28 Sonalde Desai, P. Lindsay Chase-Lansdale, and Robert Michael, "Mother or Market? Effects of Maternal Employment on the Intellectual Ability of Four-Year-Old Children," *Demography* 26 (1989): 545–61; Nazli Baydar and Jeanne Brooks-Gunn, "Effects of Maternal Employment and Child-Care Arrangements on Preschoolers' Cognitive and Behavioral Outcomes: Evidence from the Children of the National Longitudinal Survey of Youth," *Developmental Psychology* 27 (1991): 932–45.

29 NICHD Early Child Care Research Network, "Early Child Care and Children's Development Prior to School Entry" and "Further Explorations of the Detected Effects of Quantity of Early Child Care on So-cioemotional Development," both papers presented at the biennial meeting of the Society for Research in Child Development, Minneapolis, Minn., April 2001.

30 Eliana Garces, Duncan Thomas, and Janet Currie, "Longer-Term Effects of Head Start," *American Economic Review* 92 (2002): 999–1012.

31 John Love and others, *Early Head Start Research—Building Their Futures: How Early Head Start Programs Are Enhancing the Lives of Infants and Toddlers in Low-Income Families* (Princeton, N.J.: Mathematica Policy Research, 2001).

32 William Gormley and others, "The Effects of Universal Pre-K on Cognitive Development," *Developmental Psychology* 41, no. 6 (2005): 533–58.

33 W. Steven Barnett, Cynthia Lamy, and Kwanghee Jung, "The Effects of State Prekindergarten Programs on Young Children's School Readiness in Five States," *http://nieer.org/docs/index.php?DocID=129* (accessed February 13, 2006).

34 Studies relying on the ECLS-K, however, should be viewed cautiously as researchers must infer program types from parents' descriptions ("prekindergarten" may include some ordinary child care) and have limited means for adjusting for the reasons why parents select programs. The ECLS-K data also suffer from attrition of test score information over time.

35 Frances Campbell and others, "The Development of Cognitive and Academic Abilities: Growth Curves from an Early Childhood Educational Experiment," *Developmental Psychology* 37, no. 2 (2001): 231–42; Larry Schweinhart and others, *Lifetime Effects: The High/Scope Perry Preschool Study through Age 40,* Monographs of the High/Scope Educational Research Foundation 14 (Ypsilanti, Mich.: High/Scope Educational Research Foundation, 2005).

36 In studies from before 1985, the estimates might be somewhat larger because the control group had little access to alternative services. But even in the Abecedarian study by Barnett and Masse (see note 49), the control group had considerable access to center-based child care, so that change in control group experience is unlikely to have much influence on comparisons to more recent studies.

37 W. S. Barnett, "Early Childhood Education," in *School Reform Proposals: The Research Evidence,* edited by Alex Molnar (Greenwich, Conn.: Information Age Publishing, 2002), pp. 1–26.

38 Jean Larsen and Clyde Robinson, "Later Effects of Preschool on Low-Risk Children," *Early ChildhoodRe-search Quarterly* 4 (1989): 133–44.

39 Ramey, Bryant, and Suarez, "Preschool Compensatory Education" (see note 17); Martin Woodhead, "When Psychology Informs Public Policy: The Case of Early Childhood Intervention," *American Psychologist* 43 (1988): 443–54; Ron Haskins, "Beyond Metaphor: The Efficacy of Early Childhood Education," *American Psychologist* 44 (1989): 274–82; Charles Locurto, "Beyond IQ in Preschool Programs?" *Intelligence* 15 (1991): 295–312; Herman Spitz, "Commentary on Locurto's 'Beyond IQ in Preschool Programs?'" *Intelligence* 15 (1991): 327–33.

40 Frances Campbell and Craig Ramey, "Cognitive and School Outcomes for High-Risk African American Students at Middle Adolescence: Positive Effects at Early Intervention," *American Educational Research Journal* 32 (1995): 743–72; Jeanne Brooks-Gunn, Jane Waldfogel, and Wen-Jui Han, "Maternal Employment and Child Outcomes in the First

Three Years of Life: The NICHD Study of Early Childcare," *Child Development* 73 (2002): 1052–72.

41 W. Steven Barnett, "Long-Term Effects on Cognitive Development and School Success," in *Early Care and Education for Children in Poverty: Promises, Programs, and Long-Term Outcomes*, edited by W. Steven Barnett and Sarane Boocock (SUNY Press, 1998), pp. 11–44; Janet Currie, "Early Childhood Programs," *Journal of Economic Perspectives* 15 (2001): 213–38.

42 Anne McGill-Franzen and Richard Allington, "Flunk 'em or Get Them Classified: The Contamination of Primary Grade Accountability Data," *Educational Researcher* 22, no. 1 (1993): 19–22.

43 W. Steven Barnett and Greg Camilli, "Compensatory Preschool Education, Cognitive Development, and 'Race,'" in *Race and Intelligence: Separating Science from Myth*, edited by Jeff Fish (Mahwah, N.J.: Lawrence Erlbaum Associates, 2002), pp. 368–406.

44 W. Steven Barnett, John Young, and Larry Schweinhart, "How Preschool Education Influences Long-Term Cognitive Development and School Success," in *Early Care and Education for Children in Poverty*, edited by W. Steven Barnett and Sarane Boocock (SUNY Press, 1998).

45 W. Steven Barnett, "Preschool Education for Economically Disadvantaged Children: Effects on Reading Achievement and Related Outcomes," in *Handbook of Early Literacy Research*, edited by Susan Neuman and David Dickinson (New York: Guilford Press, 2001), pp. 421–43.

46 W. Steven Barnett, "Long-Term Effects of Early Childhood Programs on Cognitive and School Outcomes," *Future of Children* 5, no. 3 (1995): 25–50; Hiro Yoshikawa, "Prevention as Cumulative Protection: Effects of Early Family Support and Education on Chronic Delinquency and Its Risks," *Psychological Bulletin* 115 (1994): 27–54.

47 Arthur Reynolds and others, "Long-Term Effects of an Early Childhood Intervention on Educational Achievement and Juvenile Arrest: A 15-year Follow-Up of Low-Income Children in Public Schools," *Journal of the American Medical Association* 285 (2001): 2339–46; Dale Johnson and Todd Walker, "A Follow-Up Evaluation of the Houston Parent-Child Development Center: School Performance," *Journal of Early Intervention* 15, no. 3 (1991): 226–36; Clive Belfield and others, "Cost-Benefit Analysis of the High/Scope Perry Preschool Program Using Age 40 Follow-Up Data," *Journal of Human Resources* 41 (2006): 162–91.

48 Victoria Seitz and Nancy Apfel, "Parent-Focused Intervention: Diffusion Effects on Siblings," *Child Development* 56 (1994): 376–91.

49 W. Steven Barnett and Leonard Masse, "Comparative Benefit-Cost Analysis of the Abecedarian Program and Its Policy Implications," *Economics of Education Review* (2006, in press).

50 Garces, Thomas, and Currie, "Longer-Term Effects of Head Start" (see note 30).

51 Richard Murnane and Barbara Phillips, "What Do Effective Teachers of Inner-City Children Have in Common?" *Social Science Research* 10 (1981): 83–100; Ronald Ferguson, "Can Schools Narrow the Black-White Test Score Gap?" in *The Black-White Test Score Gap*, edited by Christopher Jencks and Meredith Phillips (Brookings, 1998), pp. 318–74; Alison Clarke-Stewart, Christian Gruber, and Linda Fitzgerald, *Children at Home and in Day Care* (Hillsdale, N.J.: Lawrence Erlbaum Associates, 1994); Carollee Howes and Michael Olenick, "Child Care and Family Influences on Toddlers' Compliance," *Child Development* 57 (1986): 202–16; Marcy Whitebook, Deborah Phillips, and Carollee Howes, *National Child Care Staffing Study Revisited: Four Years in the Life of Center-Based Child Care* (Oakland, Calif.: Child Care Employee Project, 1993); Carollee Howes, "Children's Experiences in Center-Based Child Care as a Function of Teacher Background and Adult-Child Ratio," *Merrill-Palmer Quarterly* 43, no. 3 (1997): 404–25; Leslie Phillipsen and others, "The Prediction of Process Quality from Structural Features of Child Care," *Early Childhood Research Quarterly* 12 (1997): 281–304; Barbara Bowman, M. Suzanne Donovan, and Susan Burns, eds., *Eager to Learn: Educating Our Preschoolers* (Washington: National Academy Press, 2001).

52 Harry McGurk and others, *Staff-Child Ratios in Care and Education Services for Young Children* (London: HMSO, 1995); Jean Layzer, Barbara Goodson, and Marc Moss, *Life in Preschool—Volume One of an Observational Study of Early Childhood Programs for Disadvantaged Four-Year-Olds: Final Report* (Cambridge, Mass.: Abt Associates, 1993); Susan Kontos, Carollee Howes, and Ellen Galinsky, "Does Training Make a Difference to Quality in Family Child Care?" *Early Childhood Research Quarterly* 12 (1997): 351–72; Ann Smith, "Quality Child Care and Joint Attention," *International Journal of Early Years Education* 7, no. 1 (1999): 85–98; Charles Achilles, Patrick Harman, and Paula Egelson, "Using Research Results on Class Size to Improve Pupil Achievement Outcomes," *Research in the Schools* 2, no. 2 (1995): 23–30; Harold Wenglinsky, "How Money Matters: The Effect of School District Spending on Academic Achievement," *Sociology of Education* 70, no. 3 (1997): 377–99; Fred Mosteller, "The Tennessee Study of Class Size in the Early School Grades," *Future of Children* 5, no. 2 (1995): 113–27; Jeremy Finn, Susan Gerber, and Jayne Boyd-Zaharias, "Small Classes in the Early Grades, Academic Achievement and Graduating from High School," *Journal of Educational Psychology* 97, no. 2 (2005): 214–23; Ellen Frede, "Preschool Program Quality for Children in Poverty," in *Early Care and Education for*

Children in Poverty: Promises, Programs, and Long-Term Outcomes, edited by W. Steven Barnett and Sarane Boocock (SUNY Press, 1998), pp. 77–98.

53 See Stacey Dale and Alan Krueger, "Estimating the Payoff to Attending a More Selective College: An Application of Selection on Observables and Unobservables," *Quarterly Journal of Economics* 98 (2002): 1491–527. Magnuson and Waldfogel simulate the effects on achievement from expanding early childhood education programs to clarify how wider access or upgraded preschooling can redress inequities. Expanding enrollment of black and Hispanic children to 80 percent (that is, one-third higher than the rate for white children) would close the initial gap by 4–20 percent (12–52 percent) for black (Hispanic) children. Expanding enrollments to cover all children below the poverty line would reduce the black-white (Hispanic-white) gap by at most 12 percent (16 percent). In additional simulations, upgrading all types of preschooling has no effect on gaps across ethnic groups; improving the quality of Head Start reduces racial gaps by at most 10 percent (8 percent) for black (Hispanic) children. Katherine Magnuson and Jane Wald-fogel, "Early Childhood Education: Effects on Ethnic and Racial Gaps in School Readiness," *Future of Children* 15, no. 1 (2005): 169–96.

54 Long-term health effects may be significant. Single motherhood is associated with higher rates of physical abuse and child neglect, and parental income has a strong impact on child health. See Christina Paxson and Jane Waldfogel, "Parental Resources and Child Abuse and Neglect," *American Economic Review* 89 (1999): 239–44; Anne Case, Darren Lubotsky, and Christina Paxson, "Economic Status and Health in Childhood: The Origins of the Gradient," *American Economic Review* 92 (2003): 1308–34.

55 Peter Gottschalk, "Is the Correlation in Welfare Participation across Generations Spurious?" *Journal of Public Economics* 63 (2003): 1–25; David Green and William Warburton, "Tightening a Welfare System: The Effects of Benefit Denial on Future Welfare Receipt," *Journal of Public Economics* 88 (2004): 1471–93. But the correlation may be muted, as the extent of welfare receipt scarring is debatable: scarring effects appear weak, and welfare payments are increasingly becoming time limited (most new EITC claimant families lose eligibility within two years).

56 Chris Lackey, "Violent Family Heritage, the Transition to Adulthood, and Later Partner Violence," *Journal of Family Issues* 24 (2003): 74–98.

57 Sandra Stith and others, "The Intergenerational Transmission of Spouse Abuse: A Meta-Analysis," *Journal of Marriage and the Family* 62 (2000): 640–54; Jenny Williams and Robin Sickles, "An Analysis of the Crime as Work Model: Evidence from the 1958 Philadelphia Birth Cohort Study," *Journal of Human Resources* 37 (2002): 479–509.

58 Rebecca Maynard, "The Costs of Adolescent Childbearing," in *Kids Having Kids: Economic Costs and Social Consequences of Teen Pregnancy*, edited by Rebecca Maynard (Washington: Urban Institute Press, 1996).

59 Preschooling does not have a strong effect on "steady-state" family size. It delays or reduces childbearing, by raising the opportunity cost of time spent on child care and lowering the probability of unplanned parenthood; but it raises childbearing, because of its association with higher incomes. Typically, the opportunity cost and planning effects are slightly greater than the income effect.

60 Terrie Moffitt, "Adolescence-Limited and Life-Course-Persistent Antisocial Behavior—A Developmental Taxonomy," *Psychological Review* 100 (1993): 674–701; Casey Mulligan, "Galton versus the Human Capital Approach to Inheritance," *Journal of Political Economy* 107 (1999): S184–224.

61 They also adversely influence children's test scores: being born to a teen mother reduces children's test scores at age six by 0.07 effect sizes; independently, a two-parent family is associated with test scores that are 0.1 effect size higher. See Roland Fryer and Steven Levitt, "Understanding the Black–White Test Score Gap in the First Two Years of School," *Review of Economics and Statistics* 86 (2004): 447–64.

62 Robert Haveman, Barbara Wolfe, and Elaine Peterson, "Children of Early Childbearers as Young Adults," in *Kids Having Kids: Economic Costs and Social Consequences of Teen Pregnancy*, edited by Rebecca Maynard (Washington: Urban Institute Press, 1996); Christian Belzil and Jorgen Hansen, "Structural Estimates of the Intergenerational Education Correlation," *Journal of Applied Econometrics* 18 (2003): 679–96.

63 Heather Antecol and Kelly Bedard, "Does Single Parenthood Increase the Probability of Teenage Promiscuity, Substance Abuse, and Crime?" Working Paper, University of California, *http://econ.ucsb.edu/-kelly/youth.pdf*; Cesar Rebellon, "Reconsidering the Broken Homes/Delinquency Relationship and Exploring Its Mediating Mechanism(s)," *Criminology* 40 (2002): 103–35; Jennifer Hunt, "Teen Births Keep American Crime High," Working Paper 9632 (Cambridge, Mass.: National Bureau of Economic Research, 2003).

64 Based on sixteen studies of intergenerational earnings correlations, an increase in parental income of $1,000 raises offspring income by approximately $340. See Mulligan, "Galton versus the Human Capital Approach" (see note 60). The intergenerational earnings elasticity between fathers and sons is 0.4; that is, if the father's earnings are 10 percent above the average for his generation, his son's earnings will be 4 percent higher than the average for his own generation. See Gary Solon, "Intergenerational Income Mobility in

the United States," in *Handbook of Labor Economics,* vol. 3A, edited by Orley Ashenfelter and David Card (Amsterdam: North-Holland, 1999).

65 Robert Haveman and Barbara Wolfe, "The Determinants of Children's Attainment: A Review of Methods and Findings," *Journal of Economic Literature* 33 (1995): 1829–77.

66 See Mulligan, "Galton versus the Human Capital Approach" (see note 60). Income effects on offspring attainment are similarly strong; and a two-parent family is associated with higher attainment by 0.43 years; Belzil and Hansen, "Structural Estimates" (see note 62).

67 Perry Preschool program participants had an average of 2.4 children by age forty-two. There are data on whether the first or second child has ever been arrested, repeated a grade, or been on welfare, and if the child is currently employed. There is no clear evidence of offspring advantages across these dimensions. However, sample sizes are very small.

68 Diego Restuccia and Carlos Urrutia, "Intergenerational Persistence of Earnings: The Role of Early and College Education," *American Economic Review* 94 (2004): 1354–78.

69 This result accords with other research that finds investments in youth to be less efficient than investments in young children. See Steve Cameron and James Heckman, "The Dynamics of Educational Attainment for Black, Hispanic, and White Males," *Journal of Political Economy* 109 (2001): 455–99. Our primary focus is on the efficacy of early investments *per se*, rather than on their efficacy relative to other interventions.

70 Families will have to invest resources, even if the program is publicly provided. Even with zero fees, some families do not enroll, so presumably the costs and inconvenience of enrollment must outweigh the benefits. It is possible that there is an informational problem: families do not appreciate the benefits of preschooling. However, the more likely explanation is that pre-K is not convenient for many families or that even relatively small direct expenses (such as transportation) are too much.

71 Janet Currie and Matthew Neidell, "Getting Inside the 'Black Box' of Head Start Quality: What Matters and What Doesn't," *Economics of Education Review* (2006, forthcoming).

72 W. Steven Barnett, "Maximizing Returns from Prekindergarten Education," Education and Economic Development, Federal Reserve Bank of Cleveland (November 2004), *www.clevelandfed.org/Research/Ed-Conf2004/Nov/PapersPresntns.cfm.*

11

Child Labour and Child Right to Edùcation in South Asia with Particular Reference to India and Bangladesh

Anusri Mallik

Child labour and children's rights to education have become two major issues in national development policy. Commodities produced with the help of children's labour, constitutes an important aspect of the context in which household livelihood strategies are devised and hence decisions regarding the utilization of children's labour are taken. Globalization has thrown workers in the rich industrialized countries into direct competition with workers in the poor, low-wage economies of the South Asian region and the issue of child labour has come to symbolize the politics of protectionism in the global competition for jobs. This paper focuses on the issue of child labour where the problem lies largely in the collusion between government officials, local politicians and industrialists in ensuring the perpetuation of child labour. The purpose of this paper is to explore the issue of children's right to education in the South Asian context where child labour is widely seen as a

result of massive poverty and illiteracy. An attempt has been made to draw on the experiences of India and Bangladesh to cover various themes related to the problems of universalizing education in societies marked by poverty, gender inequality, discrimination and social exclusion.

Introduction

It was five decades ago in 1959 that the United Nations (UN) General Assembly adopted the Declaration of the Rights of the Child. It was more than 25 years ago that the world celebrated 1979 as the International Year of the child, promising to herald a new framework for the welfare of the child. In 1989, world leaders became signatories to the Convention of the rights of the child. The Convention made explicit commitments on welfare and development of children defining a child as a person under the age of 18.

The question of children's needs and rights has moved into the centre stage in global debates as a result of years of activism by organizations all over the world. The adoption of a rights-based framework provides the basis for recognizing a wide range of deprivations in relation to children. It also draws attention to the enormity and complexity of the challenges ahead.

The purpose of this paper is to explore the issue of children's right to education in the South Asian context where child labour is widely seen as a result of massive poverty and illiteracy. In these countries children's economic contributions to the household sector are seen very crucial to survive their families. An attempt has been made to draw on the experiences of India and Bangladesh to cover various themes related to the problems of universalizing education in societies marked by poverty, gender inequality, discrimination and social exclusion.

Rights versus Needs

Child labour and children's rights have become major issues in the development debate around the world. A number of questions and issues have arisen and protagonists have taken diametrically opposed views on the subject, each side insisting that what they are proposing is indeed in the best interest of the child.

On the one side and more generally held, is the view that in a society where basic needs have not been fulfilled, the income of the child is important for the family's survival. This view is not widely shared. On the other side, it is often argued that poverty is a 'ruthless reality' and children have to work in order to survive. There are others, more a minority now, who believe that formal education is not necessary for the poor as it does not equip them with the apparatus of livelihood.

A recent argument which is gaining tremendous importance particularly in the non-governmental organization (NGO) sector and amongst development practitioners in the Northern World, is the belief that Children's rights must contain the right to work. Indeed there is an increasing number of people who think that children ought to be conferred on whether they want to enroll their names in school or to supply their labour in exchange of money. Listening to and acting upon children's voices has become a key issue in the United States for implementing custodial rights. It is widely believed that children should be honoured as 'full citizen' and must enjoy their rights as adults. This very act is seen as 'empowering young children to lead change' by some child right activists.

The need for education in relation to certain sections of the population include women, scheduled castes, schedule tribes and other backward classes in India is important to rectify ancient inequities in family and society. Demographers and economists have pointed to the links between female literacy, lower fertility rates and improved welfare of the society. Children have both the right to education and the need for education. Being pragmatic about the need to work and opposing the right to education, one is opposing an inter-generational perspective at all. Indeed one is falling into the trap of taking the existing reality as given. We all know that poverty is not a given phenomenon. Several factors like colonialism, capitalism, wrong government policy etc. are responsible for it. Now a-days in many countries, poverty has declined due to suitable public policy, effective public action, satisfactory economic growth rate and targeted initiatives. Even when poverty has not come down, explanations can be traced to the nature of economy and polity. People in or on the margins frequently swing to the above poverty line, though this depends to a great extent on how much below the line they originally were. Poverty then, is not static or immobile at any fixed point in time.

Child Labour and Poverty: Cause or Consequence

Does poverty cause child labour or is it child labour that causes poverty? It is an ongoing debate all over the world for more than a decade. If poverty has to be wiped out from the system, there has to be a frontal attack on child labour. Child labour is the outcome of the exploitation of the weak and underprivileged and it is always the poorest section of the society who is victimized to this exploitation. When the poor children start hard working at their young age they remain illiterate, unskilled and unable to understand and demand their rights for equal wages and better conditions of work. With their bone-breaking toils for long hours, they burn themselves out and their health is severely impaired. Like children, adults, in situations like these, are fallen heavily into debt. The rigorous circumstances of unemployment, combined with their inferior position in the society, predispose them to put their own children to work. This downward spiral of exploitation leads them to the vicious circle of poverty. Forced at an early age to accept risky works, unhygienic working conditions, long hours of work and less than minimum wages, the poor find themselves, not surprisingly, in a state of 'fake consciousness' believing that their exploiters are their patrons. Child labour therefore becomes acceptable even to those who are mostly affected by it.

So all pervasive is the belief that without upliftment of the poor, child labour cannot be stopped. The questions that are most often raised are: i) What will happen to the families of these children if child labour is stopped by law? ii) How will poor families survive without the additional earning of their children? It is seldom taken into account that income of the children is pathetically meager, and that is precisely because of the engagement of large number of children in the workforce in all the sectors of the economy. In most cases, the children are used by their parents as an asset to mortgage, when all other assets disappear.

Responsibilities of Parents

In many societies, generally, parents have been accepted as natural guardians of their children and have been presumed to work in their best interests. Parents, all over the world are seen as having 'natural rights' over their children. This right is often phrased constitutionally as a right of due process and the parent can challenge the validity of state's interference into family affairs. Pierce (1925) argued that

'The child is not the mere creature of the state; those who nurture him and direct his destiny have the right, coupled with the high duty, to recognize and prepare him for additional obligations'.[1]

But the empirical evidence from the field suggests where there are semi-feudal agrarian relations, social and economic systems are systematically put into place such as bonded labour which repeats itself over generations. Without external intrusion whether by state or community action, such arrangements would continue for an indefinite period and relationship of exploitation would remain. Children are seen by their parents as their possessions and over whom they have full right. In some societies, the duties and responsibilities of children to their parents are embedded in cultural mores and social norms. Even if there is considerable merit in the idea of parents being guardians of their children, surely the extent of their powers needs to have limits particularly when the parents themselves subscribe to the world view that children are their chattels. It is documented in several literatures as how alcoholic addiction and entertainment needs of their fathers trap them into extreme poverty and push children into work in order to sustain profligate expenditure. It is widely known how poor families inspired by consumerist boom go so far as to put their wives, daughters and sisters on prostitution within and across the borders of countries. Working women subjected to immense drudgery, both within and outside the household, often keep their girl children at home to get relief from their never-ending tasks. The greater involvement of girls in domestic and survival tasks is cited as an important reason for irregular school attendance.

The relationship between parents and children should not be seen as the property of their parents and it should be based on trusteeship. According to Arneson and Shapiro (1996), 'Children cannot be seen as chattels of their poverty and in a constitutional democracy both parents and the state have responsibilities towards the child'.[2] John Locke in his *'Two Treatises of Government'* has written extensively on parental rights and obligations. He points out that since children are not in a 'full state of equality', parents should have a sort of rule and jurisdiction over their children, and it should be a temporary one. In his words, "Because children are incapable of controlling their own conduct by their reason in a steady way that adequately caters to their prudential long-term interests and the interests of others affected by their conduct, parental obligations include the duty to govern their children".[3]

It needs to be kept in mind that, particularly in the areas of child labour, child trafficking and discrimination against the girl child, parents may not be in a position to make judgments because of cultural, social and economic reasons and therefore the state has to take certain initiatives to eliminate child labour and to include compulsory education in the larger interests of equity and good citizenship. The veil of tradition and culture is often used to mask systematic exploitation of women and children.

Educational Provision in South Asian Countries

The South Asian subcontinent consisting of the seven countries namely India, Bhutan, Nepal, Bangladesh, Pakistan, Sri Lanka and Maldives simultaneously presents a spectacle of similarities and contrasts. Almost all the countries of the region share a common history of colonialism from which they became free around 50 years ago. They therefore inherited a common administrative and educational equipment from the British colonial rulers, which continues to be a point of allusion in all discourses on educational development in the region. However, from the view point of diversities and complexities in ethnic and religious opus, political-administrative horizons, developmental policy framework as well as size and nature of the geographical territory show the countries of the region in a vastly contrasting framework.

Undoubtedly, the last five decades have witnessed momentous changes in the political and economic framework of South Asia. The most visible development, with far reaching consequence for human life, is the spread of freedom and democracy. This is of great significance as the subcontinent regions contain a population of more than a billion people that continues to burgeon at a high rate of growth. Yet, prosperity and progress in terms of improved quality of life for the people has remained tardy and unimpressive. 'Human Development Report in South Asia (2006)' has emphasized: 'The challenge for the South Asia region today is to travel the vast distance between its performance and promise. On the one hand, it has emerged as the poorest, the most illiterate, the most malnourished and the least gender-sensitive region in the world. On the other, it has all the potential to become the most dynamic region in the twenty-first century if there is massive investment in human development.' One of the most critical components of any such investment plan is 'basic education for all'.

With the exception of Sri Lanka, all the countries of South Asia began their journey towards providing mass-based education nearly half a century ago, with a huge disadvantage. In 1951, India had a literacy rate of only 16 per cent. The situation was even worse in Pakistan. Nepal began its democratization process only in 1950 and Bhutan even much later; The figures given in the tables based on the reports on human development in South Asia clearly show that except for Sri Lanka and Maldives, there is a long way to go in all the countries of the region before we can declare that all children have been brought under the fold of primary education, as the region still has around 50 million children out of school. Leaving out Sri Lanka and Maldives, adult literacy in the countries of the region remains very low ranging from 28 per cent in Nepal to 52 per cent in India.

While the aggregate position of the region paints a very dismal picture, seen from the angle of progress made by individual countries one finds certain positive developments, which hold lessons worth emulating. In fact, the variations among the countries are too vast in some respects to be bundled together for analysis.

Table 1: Literacy – Male-Female

	Adult Literacy Rate % 2006			Adult Literacy Rate % 1996		
Country	**Male**	**Female**	**Total**	**Male**	**Female**	**Total**
Bangladesh	49	26	38	47	9	24
Bhutan	56	28	42	NA	NA	NA
India	66	38	52	47	19	34
Maldives	93	93	93	NA	NA	91
Nepal	41	14	28	3	28	13
Pakistan	50	24	38	40	5	21
Sri Lanka	93	87	90	86	68	77

Source: World Development Report 2008.

Table 2: Female Enrolment

Country	Enrolment Ratios		Females as a % of Male
	1996	2006	2000-2006
Bangladesh	35	105	86
Bhutan	NA	63	61
India	56	91	82
Maldives	NA	133	97
Nepal	8	87	69
Pakistan	22	49	45
Sri Lanka	94	105	98

Source: World Development Report 2008.

Table 3: Gross Enrolment in Primary Stage

	1996			2006		
Country	Male	Female	Total	Male	Female	Total
Bangladesh	76	46	62	128	105	111
Bhutan	NA	NA	NA	82	63	73
India	98	67	83	113	91	105
Maldives	NA	NA	NA	136	133	134
Nepal	117	49	84	129	87	107
Pakistan	51	27	39	80	49	65
Sri Lanka	105	100	103	106	105	106

Source: World Development Report 2008.

Table 4: Expenditure on Education

Country	GNP per capita (% of GDP)	Expenditure on Primary Education (% of GDP)			GNP per capita (% of Annual Growth)		Current Expenditure per pupil (as a % of GNP per capita)	
	2006	1990	2000	2006	1986-1996	1996-2006	1996	2006
Bangladesh	260	1.5	2.0	2.3	- 0.3	2.7	5	6
Bhutan	390	4.2	3.7	NA	-	2.0	NA	NA
India	380	2.8	3.5	3.8	1.5	3.8	9	12
Maldives	1080	NA	9.2	8.1	-	4.1	NA	NA
Nepal	210	1.8	2.0	2.9	-	2.3	10	11
Pakistan	480	2.0	3.4	2.7	1.8	1.1	9	NA
Sri Lanka	740	2.7	2.7	3.2	2.8	3.4	9	7

Source: World Development Report 2008.

Table 5: Completion Rates and Out-of-School Children

Country	Enrolment Ratios	Females as a % of Male
Bangladesh	47	4
Bhutan	82	0.13
India	62	35
Maldives	93	NA
Nepal	52	0.97
Pakistan	48	10
Sri Lanka	98	NA

Source: World Development Report 2008.

Table 6: Number of Teachers and Pupil-Teacher Ratio

Country	Number of Teachers (ooo's)		Pupil-Teacher Ratio		Female Teachers %	
	1996	2006	1996	2006	1996	2006
Bangladesh	154	230	61	71	8	27
Bhutan	15	19	37	31	NA	16
India	156	171	61	64	27	31
Maldives	NA	NA	NA	31	NA	NA
Nepal	28	80	39	39	10	16
Pakistan	150	413	41	38	32	25
Sri Lanka	54	70	29	28	NA	82

Source: UNICEF 2008.

India: A Study

India presents a mixed picture of success and failure. On the one hand, the country has shown multifold expansion of public primary education facilities. There are nearly 700,000 schools providing primary education and more than 300,000 non-formal. Education centers and alternate schools catering to the same age group children. In terms of physical access, there is a primary school available to 93 per cent population within a distance of 1 km. Recent figures from the 61st National Sample Survey show that the national literacy rate has recorded a quick rise of 12 percentage points between 1996 and 2000. Participation of women in educational programmes has rapidly increased as compared to men than that of men. Female literacy augmented three times faster than male literacy between 1996 and 2006. Total expenditure on education (as a % of gross national product) has increased by six times from 0.7 per cent in 1980 to 5 per cent in 2006. Public expenditure on primary education as a percentage of the total education budget increased from 34.2 in 1996 to 38.5 in 2006. These incremental achievements, however, seem to be far too small for meeting the ever-expanding challenge of universal elementary education which is a constitutional commitment made five decades ago. India still accounts for 30 per cent of the total adult illiterates in the world. About 35 million children in the 6-10 years of age group do not attend primary schools.

According to the census data of 2001, around 43 per cent of the total officially registered child workers were engaged in agriculture. Around 5 per cent of the total child labour force was engaged as industrial labourer and a further 3 per cent of the total child population worked in household industry. Table 7 depicts present scenario of child labourer across major Indian states. During 2005-06, the incidence of child labour was relatively high in Andhra Pradesh, Gujarat, Karnataka, Madhya Pradesh and Rajasthan (above 8). The level was relatively low in Assam, Bihar, Haryana, Punjab and Uttar Pradesh (below 8).

Table 7: Incidence of Child Labour Across Indian States

States	NSS (2005-2006; Principal and Subsidiary Occupations)			Census 2001
	5 to 9 (rural)	10 to 14 (rural)	10 to14 (urban)	
Andhra Pradesh	2.7	24.1	0.8	13.5
Assam	0.4	5.6	0.7	4.7
Bihar	0.2	6	0.4	5.3
Gujarat	0.7	10.6	0.3	6.1
Haryana	0.1	2.6	0.2	3.5
Himachal Pradesh	0.6	8.1	0.2	4.3
Karnataka	1.1	15.3	0.6	11.2
Kerala	0	0.6	0	0.5
Madhya Pradesh	0.3	10.6	0.3	9.9
Maharashtra	0.8	8.5	0.2	8.2
Orissa	0.4	9	0.2	8.4
Punjab	0.5	5.5	0.5	3.5
Rajasthan	2.5	16.7	0.4	7.9
Tamil Nadu	0.4	8.5	0.5	5.8
Uttar Pradesh	0.2	6.5	0.6	4.3
West Bengal	0.4	8.8	0.6	4.7
India	0.7	9.3	0.4	6.5

Source: Government of India 2007.

Bangladesh: A Study

Bangladesh started with 26 per cent adult literacy rate in 1974 but it has succeeded in rapidly increasing this rate to 38 per cent by 2006. One of the major achievements of Bangladesh has been nearly wiped out gender disparity in primary enrolment. The gross enrolment ratio raised from 73 per cent in 1990 to 95 per cent in 1996. It has further been risen to 98 per cent in 2006. The net enrolment ratio has been increased to 78 per cent. The dropout rate has also been declined from 60 per cent to 40 per cent at the primary stage. The share of expenditure on primary education has been risen from an average 50 per cent to 65 per cent during the current plan period. Education expenditure as a share of total government expenditure has been increased from 9.4 per cent in the First Five Year Plan (1973-78) to 15.4 per cent during the Seventh Five Year Plan. Bangladesh has also been very successful in forging constructive partnership between the state and non-governmental organizations (NGOs) in achieving the goal of universal primary education. Table 8 sketches enrolment picture of Bangladesh. Statistical Report published by Primary and Mass Education Division reveals that enrolment of boys in primary schools has been decreased from 52.6 per cent in 2001 to 50.9 per cent in 2007. In contrast to this picture, enrolment of girls in primary schools has been increased from 47.8 per cent in 2001 to 49.1 per cent in 2007.

Table 9 describes present status of child labour in Bangladesh. According to 2006-07 CLS, child labour participation rate has been increased from 15.9 per cent in 1981-82 to 18.7 per cent in 2001-02. In between 1981-82 and 2006-07 total child population aged 10-14 years has been boosted to 17.4 million from 13.2 million. The labour force participation rate of male child was relatively high during 1981-82 to 2001-02.

Table 8: Enrolment in Primary School (2001-2007)

Year	Total (in million)	Boys (per cent)	Girls (per cent)
2001	17.2	52.6	47.8
2002	17.5	52.8	47.6
2003	18	52.8	48.1
2004	18.3	52.1	47.8
2005	17.6	51.8	48.6
2006	17.6	51.3	48.7
2007	17.6	50.9	49.1

Source: World Development Report 2008.

Table 9: Child Population and Labour Force Participation Aged 5-14 Years by Sex

Source, Period and Age Group	Total Child Population 5–14 Years ('000)			Child Labour Force 5–14 Years ('000)			Child Labour Participation Rate			Child Labour as per cent of Total Labour Force
	Both Sex	Male	Female	Both Sex	Male	Female	Both Sex	Male	Female	Both Sex
1981–82LFS*										
Total	23812	14218	13594	3782	3108	674	15.9	21.8	4.9	13.3
05–09	14563	7369	7194	608	468	140	4.2	6.3	1.9	2.1
10–14	13249	6849	6400	3174	2640	534	23.9	38.5	8.3	11.1
1986–87LFS										
Total	28316	14413	13903	3774	3098	676	13.3	21.5	4.7	12.8
05–09	14594	7387	7207	612	452	160	4.2	6.1	2.2	2.1
10–14	13722	7026	6696	3162	2646	516	23	37.8	7.7	10.7
1991-92LFS										
Total	30971	16310	14661	5979	3537	2442	19.3	21.7	16.6	11.8
05–09	19301	10123	9177	1734	1006	728	9	9.9	7.9	3.4
10–14	11671	6187	5484	4245	2531	1714	36.4	40.9	31.3	8.4
1996–97 LFS										
Total	30633	16751	13882	5923	3844	2079	19.3	22.9	15	11.6
05–09	16913	8689	8224	166	118	48	1	1.4	0.6	0.3
10–14	13720	8062	5658	5757	3726	2031	42	46.2	35.9	11.2
2001–02CLS										
Total	34455	17862	16593	6455	3856	2599	18.7	21.6	15.7	11.5
05–09	17398	8798	8600	778	440	338	4.5	5	3.9	1.4
10–14	17057	9064	7993	5677	3416	2261	33.3	37.7	28.3	10.1
2006- 07CLS#										
Total	–	–	–	–	–	–	–	–	–	–
05–09	–	–	–	–	–	–	–	–	–	–
10–14	17439	9314	8125	6777	4029	2748	38.9	43.3	33.8	11.2

* Labour Force Survey (LFS) # Child Labour Survey (CLS)

Source: World Development Report 2008.

Role of the State

In the absence of the ability of the parent to always take decisions in the 'best interests of the child', the state certainly has a role to play both for the elimination of child labour as well as for enforcing compulsory education. Without getting into an extended debate on what sort of education prepares children for the responsibilities of democratic citizenship, basic education (which goes beyond basic literacy) is needed for individuals to find spaces and make informed choices in a democratic state. Basic education is not a panacea but it does provide skills, knowledge and apparatus for the individual to negotiate spaces for himself/herself. As the judgment in 'Brown v. Board of Education, 347 US 483 493 (1954) accepted: "Today, education is perhaps the most important function of state and local governments..... it is the very foundation of good citizenship. Today, it is a principal instrument in ...... preparing (the child) for later professional training and in helping him to adjust normally to his environment."[4]

Conclusion

It is true that the Convention of the Rights of the Child, which commits the signatories to provide free education to all children, is perhaps the most authenticated international document in the world. Genuineness of the intention behind constitutional commitments and policy proclamations for guaranteeing compulsory primary education cannot be questioned. The dedication shown and the success stories presented by the civil society through non-governmental and voluntary action are quite overwhelming. Empirical evidences on opening of new educational facilities, gradually increasing public allocations for primary education in most countries of the region and enhanced support of the international community through increased financial resources, particularly, in the post-Jomtien period, are too visible to be ignored. Yet, weaning away all children even from hazardous work, getting all children into the fold of education and equipping them with basic knowledge and skills, and ensuring a safe and healthy childhood seems to be a far away goal.

(Anusri Mallik is currently working as a Faculty Associate in Icfai Research Centre, Kolkata. She can be reached at anusri.mallik@gmail.com).

Endnotes

1 'Pierce v, Society of Sisters' 268 US 510 (1925).

2 Arnesion, Richard and Ian Shapiro (1996). 'Democratic Anatomy and Religious Freedom: A Critique of Wisconsin v Yoder', in I. Shapiro (ed.), *Democracy's Place*, pp137-74 Ithaka: Cornell University Press.

3 John Locke (1680), '*Two Treatises of Government*' (Quoted in Arneson and Shapiro 1996: pp 50).

4 Brown v. Board of Education, 347 US 483 493 (1954).

References

1. Arnesion, Richard and Ian Shapiro (1996). 'Democratic Anatomy and Religious Freedom: A Critique of Wisconsin v Yoder', in I. Shapiro (ed.), Democracy's Place, pp137-74 Ithaka: Cornell University Press.
2. Basu, K. (1999), "Child Labour: Cause, Consequence and Cure with Remarks on International Labour Standards", *Journal of Economic Literature*, 37(3), 1083-1119.
3. Basu, K. and R. Ray (2002), "The Collective Model of the Household and an Unexpected Implication for Child Labour: Hypothesis and an Empirical Test", Policy Research Working Paper NO. WPS2813, World Bank, Washington (available on: *http://www.econ.worldbank.org/*)
4. Basu, K. and Z. Tzannatos (2003), "The Global Child Labour Problem: What Do We Know and What Can We Do?", *World Bank Economic Review*, 17(2), 147-174.
5. Edmonds, E. and C. Turk (2004), "Child Labour in Transition in Vietnam" in P. Glewwe, N. Agrawal and D. Dollar (ed.) *Economic Growth, Poverty and Household Welfare in Vietnam*, World Bank, Washington.
6. Emerson, P. and A.P. Souza (2003), "Is There a Child Labour Trap? Intergenerational Persistence of Child Labour in Brazil", *Economic Development and Cultural Change*, 51(2), 375-398.
7. Fyfe, A. (1989), *Child Labour*, Polity Press, Cambridge.
8. Gunnarsson, V., P.F. Orazem and M.A. Sanchez (2006), "Child Labour and School Achievement in Latin America", *The World Bank Economic Review*, 20(1), 31-54.
9. Heady, C. (2003), "The Effect of Child Labour on Learning Achievement", *World Development*, 31(2), 385-398.
10. International Labour Organisation (ILO) (2002), *Every Child Counts: New Global Estimates on Child Labour*, ILO, Geneva.

11. Jensen, P. and H.S. Nielsen, (1997), "Child Labour or School Attendance: Evidence from Zambia", *Journal of Population Economics*, 10(4), 407-424.

12. Maitra, P. and R. Ray (2002), "The joint estimation of child participation in schooling and employment: comparative evidence from three continents", *Oxford Development Studies*, 30(1), 41-62.

13. Patrinos, H.A. and G. Psacharopoulos (1997), "Family Size, Schooling and Child Labour in Peru: An Empirical Analysis", *Journal of Population Economics*, 10, 387-406.

14. Psacharopoulos, G. (1997), "Child Labour versus Educational Attainment: Some Evidence from Latin America", *Journal of Population Economics*, 10, 377-386.

15. Ray, R. and G. Lancaster (2005), "The Impact of Children's Work on Schooling: Multi-Country Evidence" *International Labour Review*, 144(2), 189-210.

16. World Development Report – Various Issues

Child Development in China

– Subhankar Dutta

China has taken The National Program of Action for Child Development (2001-2010) for the promotion of child development. Alongside the National Program, most of the provinces (99.5 percent of the counties and 97.7 percent of the districts) in China have their own policies and development plans, programs for child development. According to the National Program some policies related to the progress of child in China are: (1) try to decrease the maternal and children mortality, (2) to prevent, control and educate about the menace of HIV/AIDS, (3) to improve the education standard in extremely poor areas, (4) to protect the migrant children, (5) to protect street and homeless children, (6) to protect the girl children, (7) to punish the crimes of trafficking of women and children etc. A project titled "Safe and Healthy Growing Up Plan for Chinese Children and the Youth" (shortly, "Safe and Healthy Project") has implemented by the Chinese Children's Fund of All China Women's Federation (ACWF), targeting to help children and youth and also prevents them from drop outs, diseases, injuries and falling in crimes. In China, the literacy rate of children varies among regions. So, a nationwide policy has taken which encompasses complex management structures for nurseries (0 – 3 years), kindergartens (3 – 6 years) and preprimary classes (5 – 6 years) for enhancement of child and parent education. Also, the Chinese government has taken one of its first priority works, which relates the universal nine-year compulsory education program in poverty-stricken areas. It has already taken in reality by allocating special funds to poor and needy children for development, mainly in Western part of China. Significant number of child malnutrition in rural and poverty stricken areas of China is another concern for the Chinese government. In the Western part of China, 372 counties, largely located in remote, minority-inhabited, less developed areas lack fundamental compulsory nine-year program for education, public sanitation and other resources. The government must apply for more efforts to improve the services for its development programs in these regions. Gender bias and inequalities among children are one of the major concerns for the betterment of overall child development in the state. Stronger social and moral support and also care should be given to those children living under unfavorable conditions. Measures should also be taken to restrict the growing sex ratio, ban of illegal identification of child's sex and abortion according to parents' gender preference. Chinese government has formulated a sound legal system to care and protect the rights and interests of the development of the child. Also, Chinese government takes Action Plan (for the period of 2003 to 2010) to maintain the Polio-free status countrywide. So, as a whole China has taken a lot of programs for the development of children in the country.

(Subhankar Dutta, Research Associate, Icfai Research Centre, Kolkata. The author can be reached at subhankar@icfai.org).

References

http://www.china.org.cn/english/2005/May/130426.htm

http://www.unicef.org/china/education_child_development.html

Index

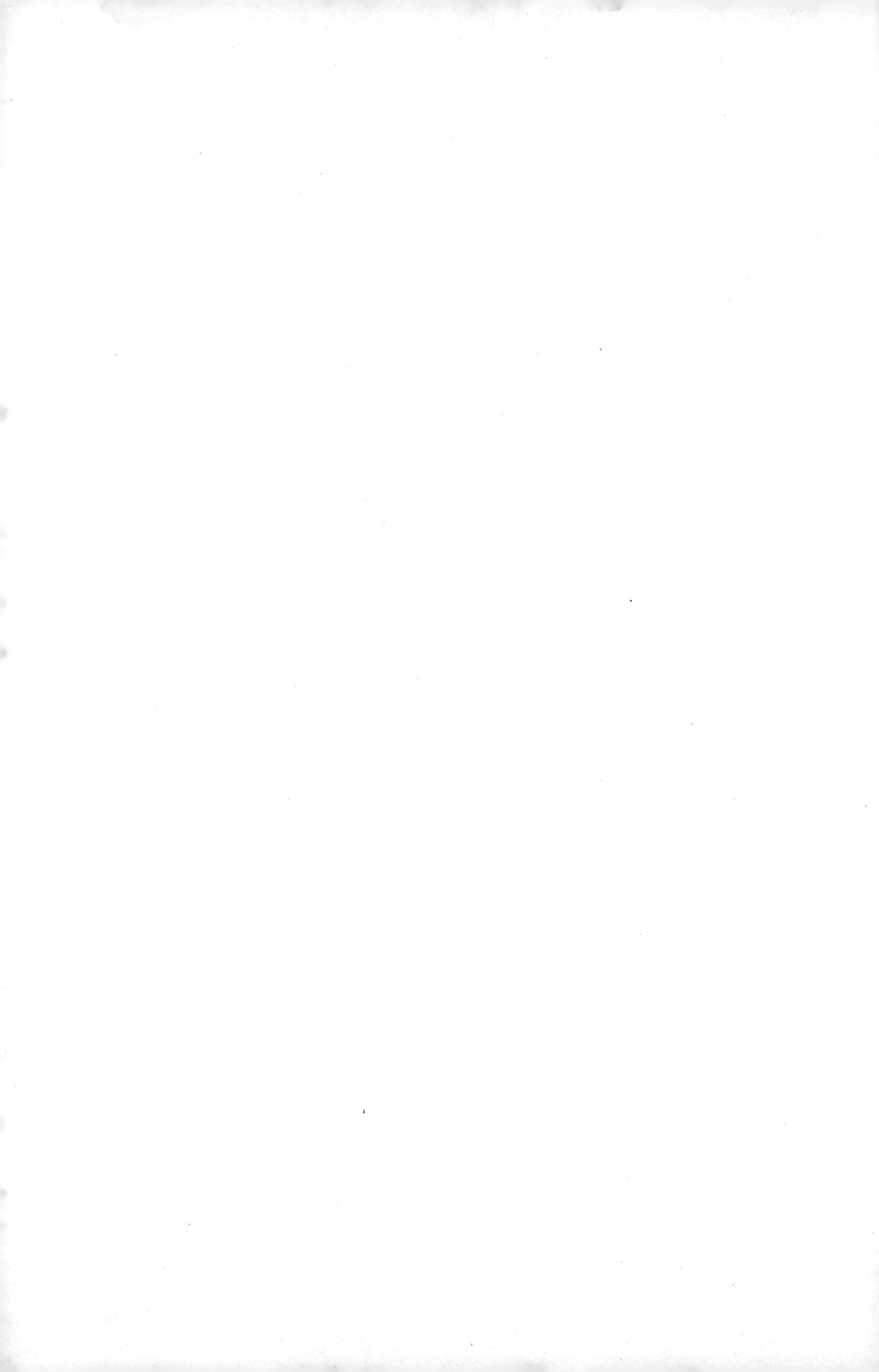